THE TOUCH THAT HEALS

THE ART OF LYMPHATIC MASSAGE

THE SECRET KEY TO STRENGTHENING
THE
IMMUNE SYSTEM

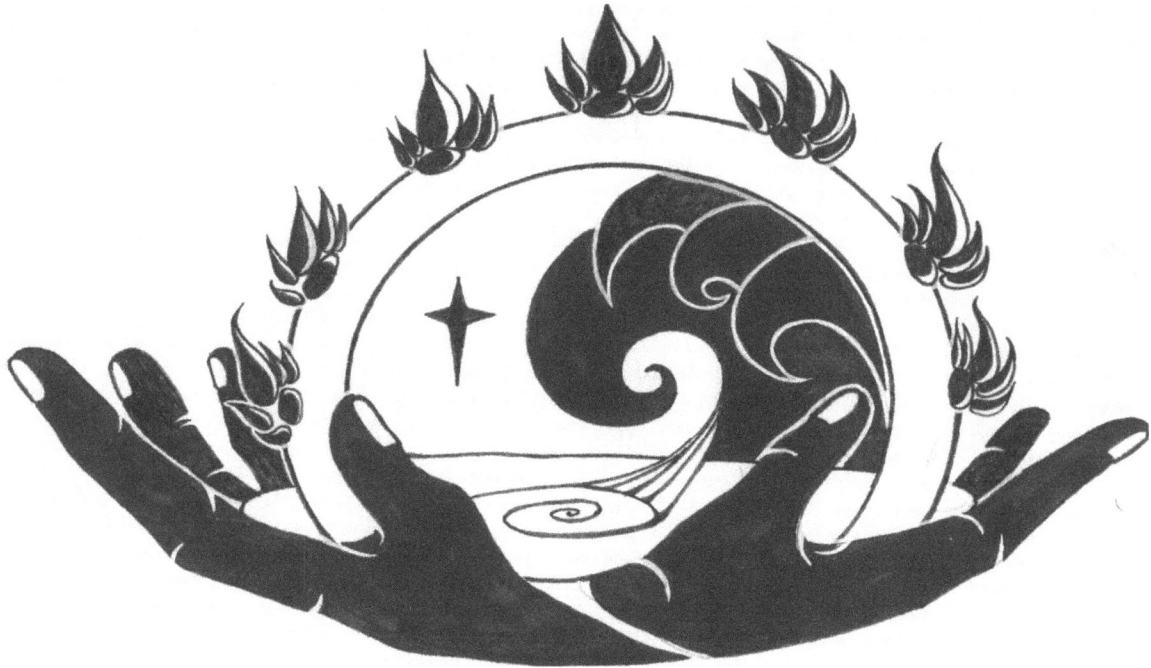

BY

DR. WILLIAM N. BROWN, Ph.D., N.D., D.Sc., L.M.T.

First printing 1995
Tal/San Publishing
Glendale, Arizona
U.S.A.

ISBN 1-884298-07-9

Second printing 2004
Revised Edition
Author House Publishing
Bloomington, Indiana
U.S.A.

ISBN 1-4184-4170-8

Third Printing 2004
Case Western Reserve University
Printing Services
Cleveland, Ohio
U.S.A.

Revised Edition 2008
Edited by Kathleen A. Scali, L.M.T.
Sedona, AZ
ISBN 978-0-615-25879-9

Available at **www.thetouchthatheals.com**

THE LYMPHATIC RAP

by

Doc (the Real Deal) Bill

Dedicated to the youth of America

Relax, unwind, get rid of the <u>static</u>
Feel the total bliss of the massage <u>lymphatic.</u>

Lymphatic will make you feel like singing and dancing
Sliding across the floor.

Make you feel so good you come back for <u>more</u>!

Babies and mothers and grandparents <u>too</u>
Say lymphatic massage makes you feel brand <u>new</u>!

Strengthen the immune system,
***Rejuvenate** the <u>cells.</u>*

Feel young again, healthy and <u>well</u>.

Accelerate the lymph stream
Quicken the <u>spirit</u>!

It's the power of the universe
Bringing you near to <u>it</u>.

Lymphatic fights colds, viruses, even the <u>flu</u>.

Lymphatic massage is good for <u>you</u>!

So experience white light vortex <u>energy</u>
And you will feel as good as can <u>be</u>.

Very, very healthy and totally stress <u>free</u>!

So listen to the word and make sure
You hear <u>it</u>.

Lymphatic heals your mind, body and <u>spirit</u>.

This is the truth <u>folks</u> and you need to <u>know</u>, Lymphatic is the healing touch
That is better than <u>dope</u>!

This book is dedicated

To my grandmother, **Rev. Mabel Smith, Ph.D.**,

and to the **GREAT MASTER** to whom this work honors.

TABLE OF CONTENTS

PART THREE

PART FOUR

PART FIVE

THE FOUNDATION FOR HOLISTIC HEALTH THERAPY
William N. Brown, Ph.D.
20475 Farnesleigh Rd., suite #111
Shaker Hts., OH 44122
(216) 254-7368 USA

September 21, 1988

C. Everett Koop, M.D., Surgeon General
The Public Health Service
Office of the Assistant Secretary for Health
200 Independence Avenue, Southwest
Washington, D.C.   20201

Dear Dr. Koop:

I applaud your dedication and diligent efforts to change the lifestyle of Americans in an attempt to raise the overall health quotient of America. Your substance abuse programs (tobacco, alcohol, and drugs), and your leadership in this area is appreciated by those of us dedicated health care professionals who share in your goals. However, in the area of medical massage therapy, there are thousands of qualified professionals whose skills are underutilized due to a lack of knowledge on the part of medical professional as to the efficacy of massage therapy.

Recent television interviews with medical experts specializing in the field of Multiple Sclerosis, stated that they had no knowledge of any massage or massage technique that had any effect whatsoever on Multiple Sclerosis. There is long standing medically documented evidence to the contrary. Massage is a legitimate, therapeutic procedure and may be of help to people suffering from Multiple Sclerosis. These procedures cannot reverse the disease, but give support to the muscular, circulatory, and lymphatic systems of the body and can provide some symptomatic relief.1

More specifically, lymphatic massage therapy may also be of great benefit due to the autoimmunogenic aspect of the disease by addressing the immune system directly through lymphatic massage therapy.2 Research on lymphatic massage therapy has also been done in Jerusalem, Israel at The Vascular Clinic, Hadassah Hospital, Televiv Medical Center by Professor F.G. Sulman.

Furthermore, there are many other fields of preventative and health maintenance care where licensed, medically trained and approved individuals are not being utilized. Caesarean neonatal care is one specific instance. Death from respiratory disorders is 10 times more frequent in Caesarean delivered babies than in vaginally delivered babies. This higher incidence of fatality may be due to the lack of natural massage which occurs during passage through the birth canal.3   Massage techniques scientifically utilized in a specific approach call infant massage, could greatly reduce the instance of respiratory dysfunction with a great savings of life and money.

There are many other areas where licensed medical massage therapists can and should be used in the maintenance of health. The health concerns of older Americans can also be addressed through medical massage therapy. In Geriatric care, improved circulation, immune stimulation and increased nutrition are critical factors, all of which are a direct result of therapeutic medical massage. Clearly, massage is important from birth to our twilight years in the maintenance and preservation of our health.

I am writing this letter to you, Dr. Koop, because I am impressed with your farsighted dedication to the improved health of America. I hope these suggestions and references are of help.

Very truly yours,

William N. Brown, Ph.D.

WNB/mlh

1. *The Art of Massage*; John Harvey Kellogg, M.D., LL.D., F.A.C.A.; Modern Medicine Publishing Co.; Battle Creek, Michigan; 1929; page 46.

2. *Manual of Dr. Vodder's Lymph Drainage*; Ingrid Kurtz, M.D.; Haug Publishers; Heidelberg; 1986; pages 97-98.

 3. *Touching, the Human Significance of the Skin*; Ashley Montague, Ph.D.; Harper & Row, Publishers; New York; 1986; pages 61-64.

DEPARTMENT OF HEALTH & HUMAN SERVICES   Public Health Service

_____

National Institutes of Health
Bethesda, Maryland 20892
Building : 1
Room   : 258
(301) 496-   6614

October 14, 1988

William N. Brown, Ph.D.
The Foundation for
  Holistic Health Therapy
11750 Shaker Boulevard
Suite 108
Cleveland, Ohio 44120

Dear Dr. Brown:

This is in response to your letter of September 21, addressed to
Surgeon General C. Everett Koop, in which you point out that due
to a lack of public and professional knowledge there is an under
utilization of "medical massage therapy."

You are no doubt correct in assuming that there is gross under
utilization of massage therapy in the United States, due to the
fact this has not been an area of emphasis in our health
maintenance systems. As you state, massage therapy is an
important adjunct toward the maintenance and preservation of our
health "from birth to our twilight years," and therefore should
be applied on a more routine basis.

Upon consulting with experts on multiple sclerosis in the
National Institute of Neurological and Communicative Disorders
and Stroke, it was stated they are not aware of any scientific
evidence that documents the value of massage in the management of
multiple sclerosis. But as you indicate, on an individual basis
massage therapy "may be of help to people suffering from multiple
sclerosis."

In regard to cesarean birth you are correct that there is an
increased incidence of respiratory disorders. As reported in
most retrospective studies, cesarean birth, independent of
maternal complications, appears to be associated with a
increased incidence of respiratory distress at all gestational
ages. The overall conclusion from many epidemiological and
experimental studies is that birth by cesarean in the absence of
labor results in a higher incidence of respiratory distress
syndrome (RDS). It is not clear, however, that the more frequent
respiratory distress is due to RDS. It is clear, however, that
the increased respiratory distress contributes to clinical
morbidity. Ill-timed cesarean birth continues to occur and
should be preventable, and therefore, it is recommended that the
guidelines on timing of cesarean birth should be followed as

outlined in the 1979 document of the American College of
Obstetricians and Gynecologists and the American Academy of
Pediatrics.

Obviously, more research is needed to explain the effects of
labor, the altered hormonal environment associated with labor,
the effects of thoracic compression during vaginal delivery, and
the effects of anesthesia on neonatal physiology. It should be
emphasized that in infants born at or near term with demonstrably
mature lungs, respiratory distress is unlikely to be a problem
whatever the route of delivery.

As you well appreciate, the field of medicine and health is a
complex and difficult one that requires the dedication of
individuals from diverse and varied fields, and there is no
question that the Foundation for Holistic Health Therapy, and the
application of medical massage therapy, should be a part of those
efforts.

Thank you for sharing your views and we are appreciative of your
interests in the efforts of the Public Health Service.

Sincerely,

John T. Kalberer, Jr., Ph.D.
Deputy Director, Division of
Disease Prevention

cc: William T. Friedewald, M.D.

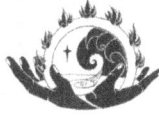

Dr. William N. Brown, N.D., Ph.D.

Naturopathic Center
20475 Farnsleigh Rd., #111
Shaker Hts., Ohio 44122
(216) 254-7368

December 26, 2003

To: The Honorable Nelson Mandela
From: Dr. William Brown, Ph.D., N.D.

Dear Mr. Mandela:

I am Dr. William N. Brown, Ph.D., N.D. I work as a naturopathic health care practitioner in Shaker Heights, Ohio, U.S.A. I am writing to you because I admire and respect the courageous stand you have taken in your heroic attempt to help the people of South Africa who are suffering with AIDS, and other immune deficiency syndromes.

I teach a natural method of healing that strengthens the immune system. It is a simple technique that can be learned in as little as (3) three days. I have practiced this method for almost (20) twenty years with great success. There is an abundance of research that demonstrates the effectiveness of this work. I would like to some to South Africa to teach this method to as many people that would want to learn how to make the immune system stronger. My work and some of my experiences with this method are in my book **THE TOUCH THAT HEALS.**

I humbly offer my services to you and the people of South Africa in an honest attempt to help improve the quality of life for those that are afflicted with this terrible disease. May God keep you strong and bless you with clear vision to continue to lead the people of South Africa to a better and healthier life in years to come.

Thank you for your kind attention to this letter of request to be of service.

With Light and Love,

William N. Brown, Ph.D., N.D.
Imhotep Aten Amen-Ra

x

Dr. William N. Brown
60 Buena Vista Lane
Sedona, Az 86336

March 21, 2008

Senator Barack Obama
713 Hart Senate Office Building
Washington, D.C. 20510

John C. Kluczynski Federal Office Building
230 South Dearborn St.
Suite 3900 (39th floor)
Chicago, Illinois 60604

Dear Senator Obama:

I am writing you this letter because you stated in your health care program that a great emphasis would be placed on preventative health care. I am a Doctor of Nutrition, Naturopath and Licensed Massage Therapist, specializing in lymphatic massage; a profoundly gentle massage technique that demostratively strengthens the immune system. The question I have for you a this time is: How have you implemented preventative health care in your own life?

Natural preventative health care is my speciality. Lymphatic massage stimulates and makes the immune system strong with all the attendant benefits of a strong immune system; i.e., no illness or less severity or less duration of illness. This technique, while used in the traditional medical model that is after trauma and surgery its efficacy has been demonstrated. However, the use of this procedure as a preventative measure is little known in the medical community.

I am offering to provide this specialized form of preventative health care service to you and your family to help maintain your health while during your ardgeous campaign. Being exposed to large crowds, recycled air on airplanes, lack of sleep and stress may compromise the immune system at a time when you need your strength the most.

I have lectured on this procedure and its benefits at Case Western Reserve University's School of Medicine and I train licensed massage therapists in this procedure. So for God's sake, please allow me to either provide the treatments for you and your family or allow me to train someone you designate so that this procedure may be of service to you and be more fully implemented in the health care of America.

If massage therapists all over America were trained in lymphatic massage, as a preventative health care measure, you and others would be able to obtain services wherever you may be and thereby significantly reduce health care costs for all. The National Institute of Health, Bethesda, MD, in their response to my communication, acknowledged the preventative health benefits of lymphatic massage on the immune system but did not use the procedure because physical medicine was not their emphasis.

Of course, the ideal would be for the health insurance industry to provide coverage for preventative health care services such as lymphatic massage and other proven alternative health care procedures. Currently medical doctors do not give written prescriptions to massage therapists for lymphatic massage, they do give them to physical therapists who do not do massage, apparently due to insurance and medicare guidelines. These guidelines are denying preventative health care to millions of Americans as well as impacting the livlihood of thousands of licensed health care professionals.

If you have a structured preventative health care plan for yourself and your family, is it through your congressional health care plan and does it cover lymphatic massage and/or massage?

Thank you for all you have done and are yet to do for the good of all Americans. I hope you will allow me to help you in your quest for better health care in America.

Very truly yours,

The Foundation for Holistic Health Therapy

Dr. William N. Brown

PREFACE

"Where touching begins, there love and humanity also begin---"

Dr. Ashley Montague

Until now, I have been unable to find a definitive work on the history, technique, and practice of Lymphatic Massage. So after fifteen years as a practitioner of this ancient, gentle and effective art, I have decided to write. I have divided this work into five sections.

Part One is for those who have never heard of Lymphatic, as Manual Lymph Drainage or as Lymphatic Massage. I hope that this is informative to people who desire a better understanding of the nature and function of the immune system.

Part Two contains the lymphatic massage procedure and RamaChi, or self help Lymphatic Massage, with detailed instruction and photographs. This is a unique combination of TaiChi and Lymphatic Massage. Part Three contains some anecdotal case histories from my practice.

Part Four is for therapists and other dedicated professionals who desire to broaden their knowledge so they may be of greater service to others. Part five offers classes, video tapes, and further instruction in the art of Lymphatic Massage.

There are many thousands of people who suffer from chronic disease of an immune dysfunction origin. This technique of Lymphatic Massage will help immensely. It is my intention that the knowledge of this profound yet simple procedure will be shared by people in America and throughout the world. It is my prayer that the many thousands of people who now exist in the darkness of pain, may know the joy of healing in the love and light of Lymphatic Massage.

Goethe said: "Magnetism is an all-present, all reaching power. Every human being has it. Only according to the human individuality it differs in strength. Its action works on everything and magnetism is everywhere." We do not have to doubt any longer that a power leaves our hands. The Kirlian photography shows and proves that.

The electro-magnetic forcefield is **not** the only energy which can be employed and used for healing. There is the Prana Energy. An energy which penetrates each cell of our body and flows from East to West. To work on the development of your light within you is to realize the power of lymphatics. In the basic technique of lymph massage, the focus is to channel white light and experience personal and universal energy.

It is important you understand this book is a textbook for lymphatic massage, which makes use of the tremendous electro-magnetic power of the universe.

The entire body of man is a field flowing electro-magnetic energy. Where ever this flow stops, for one reason or another, we have a short circuit and the pattern of life and health is impaired.

Lymphatic massage, done in the right manner, may aid in bringing back the energy and full flow and repair the "the short circuit" and health is restored. To obtain full mastery of the lymphatic massage, one has to know the exact manner and flow of the human lymphatic system and biomagnetic energy patterns. [See Figs. 1(a) and 1(b)]

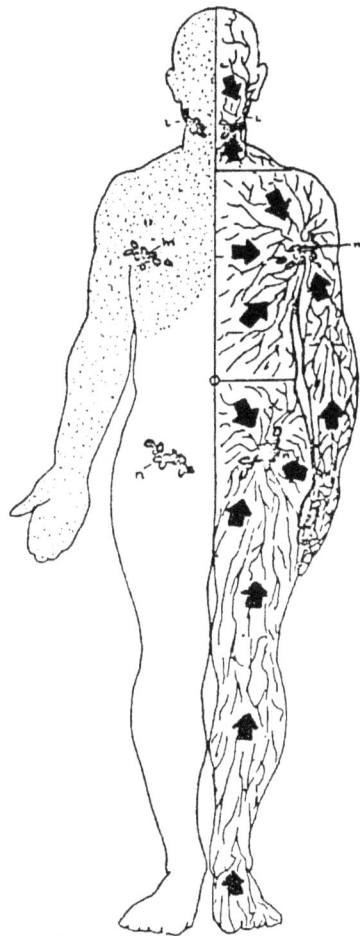

Fig. 1(a)

THE LYMPHATIC ELECTROMAGNETIC COMPOSITE PICTURE OF THE
PATTERN FORCES OF THE BODY AND THEIR WIRELESS CIRCUITS

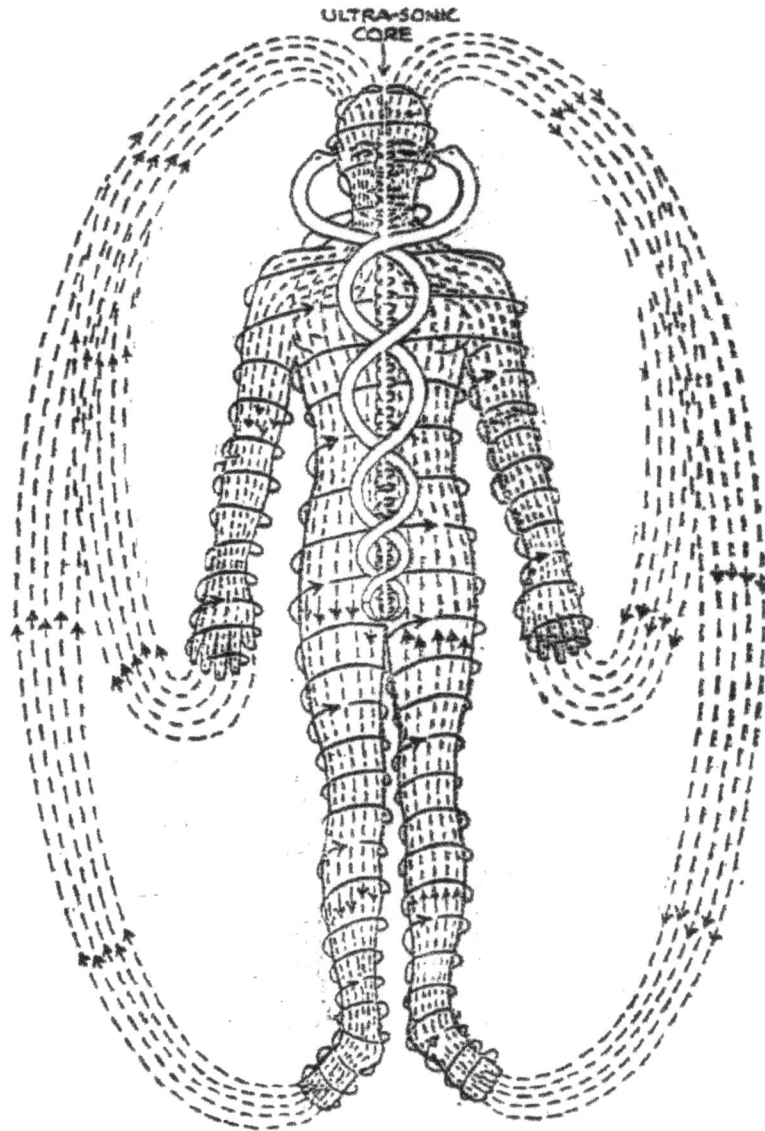

Fig. 1(b)

INTRODUCTION

The Origins, History and Development of Lymphatic Massage

To discover the true beginning of lymphatic massage, one must examine the healing practices of Ancient Egypt. Lymphatic massage was developed from the humoral therapy (See Fig. 2) as practiced by the true Father of Medicine, Imhotep. Imhotep (2640 BC) was a doctor, architect, high priest, scribe and adviser to Pharaoh Netjerikhet/King Djoser. His name means "the one that comes in peace."

Imhotep was the high priest of Heliopolis, which was the religious capital of Egypt. He practiced the ancient humoral therapy in his school of medicine at Memphis, known as the Cult of Askepion. It is said that Imhotep was taught by Tuhati (African name), who the Greeks called Thoth the Atlantean. Thoth was the wisest of the Egyptian Gods. He overcame the curse of RA and helped Isis to bring Osiris back from the dead. Thoth was the eloquent messenger of the Gods and especially Tfnut, Lunar Goddess of water, which relates specifically to the humoral therapy from which lymphatic massage is derived.

Humoral therapy can be regarded in the category of medical science since it explains the causes of many diseases and suggests ways of treatment and prevention. According to the Edwin Smith Papyrus written C. 1700 BCE, the teachings of Imhotep, predate the major humoral traditions of the Hippocratic-Galenic (or Graceo-Persian-Arab), the Ayurvedic of India and the Chinese by a thousand years. He had a through knowledge of the circulatory system and he also used vibrational color therapy with focused beams of light and gem stones combined with spiritual prayer and humoral therapy (lymphatic massage) to eradicate illness. Sadly, knowledge of these procedures were lost, perhaps when the library at Alexandria was burned and much ancient knowledge was lost. The Greeks, who gained their knowledge from Egypt, were unaware of many of the subtle methods used for healing. Hippocrates (460-377BC) describes a lymphatic temperament, however, the anatomy and physiology of the lymphatic system were not empirically determined until the 17th Century.

- In 1622, Gaspard, Asselli (1581-1626), an Italian physician, discovered the "milky veins" of a dog after digestion. This is documented as the first historical discovery of the lymphatic vessels.

   We can note that shortly afterwards in England, 1628, William Harvey published his discoveries about the systemic blood circulation.

- In 1650-51, John Pecquet (1622-1674) from Dieppe, France, described the lymphatic duct, the largest lymphatic vessel of the body", and its unique beginning in the "Cysterna Chyli" or "Pecquet's cystern."

Time c. 3000-1700 BCE

Title Imhotep and the Edwin Smith Papyrus

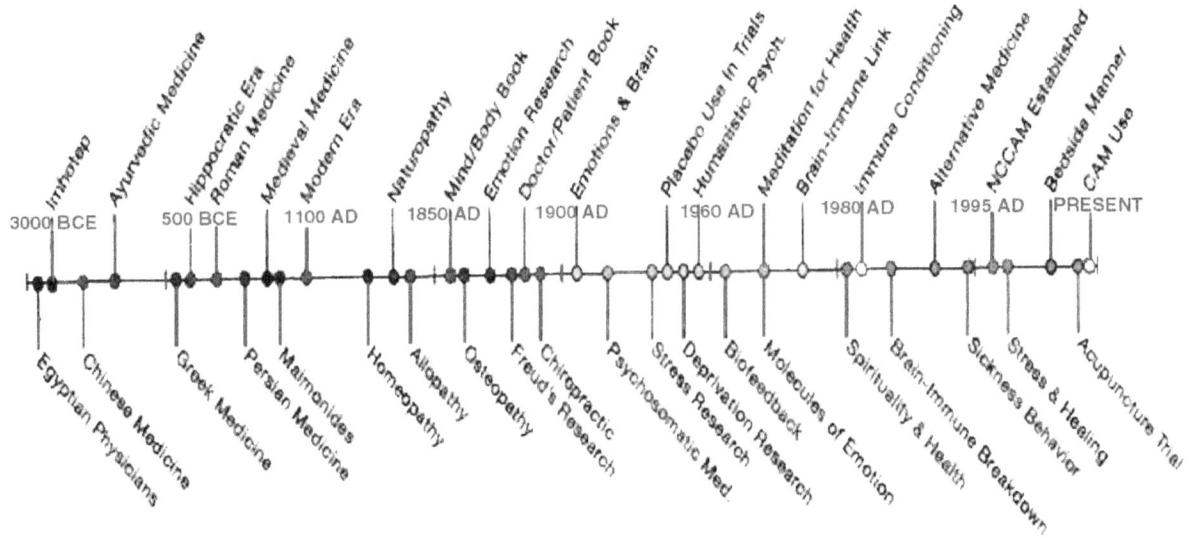

Event A seminal compilation of Egyptian medical practice, now called the Edwin Smith Papyrus, is written c. 1700 BCE based on the teachings of the Egyptian physician Imhotep who lived around 2640 BCE.

Imhotep is considered a founder of ancient Egyptian medicine. He performed surgeries and used established methods for examining, diagnosing, and treating patients. Like other healers during this time, spiritual beliefs were an important part of his practice.

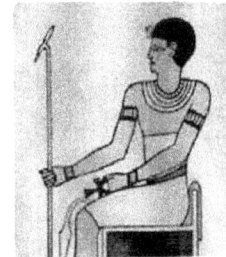

Egyptian god Imhotep.

The Papyrus itself is named after an American living in Cairo who purchased it in 1862. Smith also purchased another important medical papyrus, the Ebers Papyrus that includes medical information dating back as far as 3000 BCE.

Successful treatments for mental health are usually attributed to the kindness of a patron god or to the power of an amulet. However, some mental health treatments resemble modern methods, including sleep and occupational therapies.

Medical writings discuss body anatomy in detail and contain the first descriptions of the brain. They also mention the heart, liver, spleen, kidneys, bladder and blood vessels. Blood vessels are believed to carry air or mucus. Two vessels flowing to the right ear are thought to contain the breath of life, and two to the left ear the breath of death.

Healers are also priests. Different priests specialize in different parts of the body, much like modern doctors specialize today. Egyptians believe that different gods govern different sectors of the human body.

Fig. 2

- 1652 Bartholins designated the term lymph for the clear body water.

- Olauf Rudbeck (1630-1708) was a scientific genius from Sweden Uppsala). He was the first anatomist to see and consider the lymphatic as a complete and specific system in the human body that could be compared to the venous circulation. He can be referred to as the first man who truly discovered the lymphatic system, and understood it as a whole system.

- Sappey - Anatomy of the lymphatic system - 1874

- Alexander of Winiwarter (1848-1910), a surgeon from Belgium, was the first physician to introduce an effective protocol using manual techniques (heavy pressure) in hospitals for draining lymphedemas.

- F.P. Millard, Canadian osteopath, founder and president of the International Lymphatic Society, editor of a quarterly journal published by the Lymphatic Research Society, proposed a new osteopathic technique of "diagnosing various disease by palpating lymphatic glands." In Applied Anatomy of the Lymphatics, 1922, he used the term "lymphatic drainage," and suggested different lymphatic drainage techniques to affect the lymphatic flow.

- Emil Vodder (1896-1986), a Danish massage practitioner, and doctor in philosophy (1928), had further intuition, an inspired insight, to drain the lymph of one of his patients that suffered from chronic, sinusitis and diffuse acne. This took place between 1932 and 1936 in Cannes, French Rivera, in his physiotherapeutical institute. He further developed, for the first time, a precise manual technique for lymph drainage. Initially, he began to reveal and demonstrate this technique in cosmetogical congresses throughout Europe (beginning with Paris, 1936)

- In 1946 Dr. Johannes Asdonk, M.D. of Essen stated that in his medical practice, all cases of local lymph stagnation and consequential under nutrition of the tissues responded perfectly to lymph drainage. Dr. Askonk helped to establish a clinic with Dr. Vodder in Germany in 1973.

- In 1963, A. J. Barth in Munich Germany, a volume containing 43 theses on the lymphatic system and lymphatism was produced by a team of scientists under the leadership of Dr. Max Josef Zilch, M.D.

In the year 1932, a Danish physio-therapist and massage practitioner by the name of Emil Vodder, through intuition inspired insight, was led to do circular motions over swollen lymph vessels of patients that came to him in the French Rivera. He further developed this technique for manual lymph drainage with Dr. Johannes Asdonk. Together they established a clinic in the Black Forest in German where they developed a precise manual technique for lymph drainage.

In the 1936 Beauty and Health Exhibition in Paris, Dr. Vodder demonstrated his basic technique to the cosmetologic congress throughout Europe, which created a revolution in skin therapy. The establishment of the Society for Dr. Vodder's Manuel Lymph Drainage, and the recognition of MLD by the National Health Insurance schemes in 1972 was a two edged sword as the complete systems of lymph drainage was reduced to a piece meal approach. The cost restraining law of the National Health Insurance required this fracturization of the technique and reduced it to a physical therapy and moved lymph drainage away from a full body massage technique. Dr. Vodder stated in his commentary on the technique of manual lymph drainage:

> We should now like to deal with the whole body treatment. We Masseurs are not unacquainted with complete treatment and medical care even if we are compelled to carry out many partial treatments. In apology we say that reflexes brought about by the treatments do indeed have an impact on the "whole person" when whole body drainage is performed we directly influence 50%of the total connective tissue in the body!

It is clear that Dr. Vodder is stating unequivocally that the whole body is superior. It is also very clear that as a result of governmental insurance schemes and the subsequent alternation of the technique of manual lymph drainage, the concept of systemic acceleration of the flow of the lymph stream has been lost due to the practice of many partial treatments. Furthermore, the technique itself was changed, omitting crucial and key elements of the technique. Now, 36 years later (1972-2008), very few practitioners are aware of the enhanced, increased and complete effect of the accelerated flow of the lymph stream systemically (throughout the entire system) including organs, vessels, capillaries and cells, which is faciliated by the complete approach to the full body treatment. The complete system that Dr. Vodder taught originally has been preserved by his "golden hands" student Dr. Annie Childs.

Dr. Childs studied with Dr. Vodder in Paris, London in1965 and with Vodder and Asdonk in Saigerhoh Klinik in the Black Forest region of Germany in 1973. (See Fig. 3) At that time, the original technique was still being taught. After the national insurance required the break up of the original technique very few still know the original technique and its essential elements.

I have studied with Dr. Annie Childs and with Hildegard Whittlinger, Director of the Vodder School in Austria (See Fig. 3-A and 3-B). I have practiced the lymph massage since being trained by Dr. Childs in 1982. Since I have studied with both instructors, I am aware of the essential differences in the full body approach and the piece meal approach which omits key elements which would enhance and improve the piece meal approach. These key elements which I have named the Advanced Lymphatic Protocols for Manual Lymph Drainage, reintegrate these lost key elements, which can be applied to any form or style of lymph drainage and facilitate the complete flow of the system which was lost by the change in 1972. (See Fig. 4)

Lymphdrainage-Grundkurse

Herbst 1973/74

Kursleiter: Dr. Emil Vodder und Frau Estrid Vodder

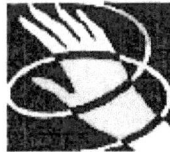

DR. VODDER KLINIK
SAIGERHÖH
staatlich anerkannt
beihilfefähig

Chefarzt: Dr. med. JOHANNES ASDONK

7821 SAIG / Titisee / Südl. Hochschwarzwald

Bahnhof Titisee · Fernruf 07653 / 741 · Telex 07722314

Heilverfahren:

Manuelle Lymphdrainage und Chirotherapie

mit Diagnostikabteilung (Röntgen, Enzymlabor, Ekg.)
Bäderabteilung f. Kneipp'sche und mediz.-physikal. Therapie
Hallenbad, Sauna, Solarium
Tennishalle und Tennisplätze
Waldreiches Schonklima in 1000 m ebener Höhenlage
Geeignet auch für Kreislaufschwache

Heilanzeigen:

Lymphoedem der Arme und Beine

Rehabilitation und Rekonvaleszenz

nach Unfällen, bei Sudeck'scher Dystrophie
nach inneren Erkrankungen, Herz- und Kreislaufleiden u.ä.
nach Hals- Nasen- Ohren- Krankheiten
bei nervöser Erschöpfung
nach Apoplexien

Krampfaderbeinleiden, hartnäckige Beingeschwüre u.a.

Kopfschmerzleiden, Trigeminusneuralgien, Migräne u.a.

Wirbelsäulenschmerzen, Ischialgien, Neuralgien

Gelenk- und Muskelrheumatismus

Lymphatische und entwicklungsgestörte Kinder mit Begleitperson

Fig. 3

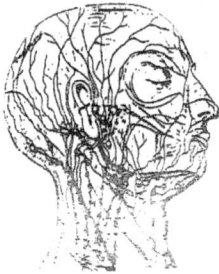

Dr. Anita Childs Ph.D.
Lymphatic Manipulation Center
Holistic Healthology Center
1381 Callens Rd.
Ventura, Ca. 93003
ph. 805-653-1555

Dear Students: Nov. 24th /86.

This is an invitation to all of my students for a review
of your lymphatic manipulation technique to make sure that it
is being done correctly. I want to make sure there are no
imperfections in your manipulation. The fee is $30.00. Cash only

A celluite treatment class will be given after the lymphatic
manipulation review. The cost of the class is $100.00 .Cash only

I hope to hear from you soon.

                          Sincerely,

Date of classes Dec./86 , 6th +7th., the 13th + 14th.. the 20th + 21 th.

Time 10AM to 6 PM.   Dr. Anita Childs, PH.D.

Dr. Anita Childs Ph.D.
Lymphatic Manipulation Center
Holistic Healthology Center
1381 Callens Rd.
Ventura, Ca. 93003

Fig. 3-A

Fig. 3-B

Manual Lymph Drainage

BASIC COURSE

INSTRUCTOR:
Hildegard Wittlinger
from the
Dr. Vodder School
in Walchsee, Austria

COURSE COORDINATOR:
Dana L. Wyrick, R.M.T.
Certified Lymph Drainage Therapist

Introduction to Dr. Vodder's Manual Lymph Drainage

Volume 3: Therapy II
(Treatment Manual) By Ingrid Kurz MD

Translated by

Robert H. Harris HND (Appl. Biol. U.K.)

■ Manual Lymph Drainage is a Massage Technique developed in the 1930's by Dr. Emil Vodder, a European Physical Therapist.

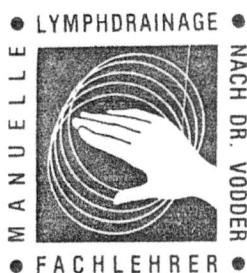

■ Manual Lymph Drainage has been researched over the last 20 years by such scientists as, M. Foldi, E. Kuhnki, and others. It's physiological benefits are well documented.

■ Manual Lymph Drainage is covered by Government Health Plans in various countries in Europe, consequently it is prescribed by physicians and practiced in hospitals.

■ Manual Lymph Drainage is a precise technique designed to promote the normal functioning of the lymphatic system. It is used primarily in the treatment of edematous tissue and various chronic inflammatory conditions. Manual Lymph Drainage facilitates the removal of metabolic wastes, excess water, toxins, bacterium, viruses, broken cells, plasma proteins, large fat molecules and foreign substances from the tissues via the lymphatic vessels and venous capillaries. Therapeutic application of Manual Lymph Drainage enhances the activity of the immune system, reduces pain, and stimulates the parasympathetic nervous system.

Hildegard Wittlinger is world renown as a Lecturer and Teacher of Manual Lymph Drainage. Mrs. Wittlinger has taught in North America, Central America, Europe and Africa. Along with her husband, Gunther, Mrs. Wittlinger directs the famous Dr. Vodder School in Walchese, Austria. The school has been in operation for 20 years and is the recognized authority of the Dr. Vodder method. In 1981 Dr. Vodder appointed the Wittlingers his successors.

COURSE DATES:	July 11 through 15, 1986 (Fri.–Tues.)
LOCATION:	Kikkawa College 3 Riverview Gardens Toronto, Ontario, Canada M6S 4E4 (416) 762-4857
COST:	$450 (Canadian)
PREREGISTRATION FEE:	$50 (Canadian) The preregistration fee is due prior to June 15th, 1986. This is a non-refundable fee and will be applied to your tuition fees. Cheques should be made payable to the Kikkawa College and sent to the College address along with the registration form.

For additional information call Kikkawa College (416) 762-4857

LECTURE FOR PHYSICIANS AND HEALTH CARE PROFESSIONALS

Translator Note
Manual Lymph Drainage ad modum Vodder
Its Theory and Therapeutic Effects
Speaker: Hildegard Wittlinger

This book was translated by *Robert H. Harris* HND, (Appl. Biol., U.K.), who is a registered massage therapist in Toronto, Canada, and specializes in manual lymph drainage therapy.

The Advanced Lymphatic Protocols now allow for the re-integration of the lost elements of lymph massage. No matter what system one may practice, i.e. French, German, partial or full body treatments, the Advanced Lymphatic Protocols will dramatically improve your results with the benefit of a more effective treatment which ultimately benefits the health of your patients.

Lymphatic can be a self transformational technique; an experiential development of the integration of self and cosmos. Without this connection, the practice is limited to a mere technique rather than a healing. Lymphatic massage allows for the movement of the soul to an epiphany in both practitioner and patient. To obtain full mastery of lymphatic massage, lymphatic movement of the system must include the introduction of TiaChi and energy, elevating lymphatic massage to an evolutionary self realization process.

Lymphatic massage is the art of the formless form. One does not intellectualize, but rather experiences the macro and micro aspects of universal energy of lymphatic massage through practice; and through practice, comes understanding and mastery!

We are made in the image of the universe.

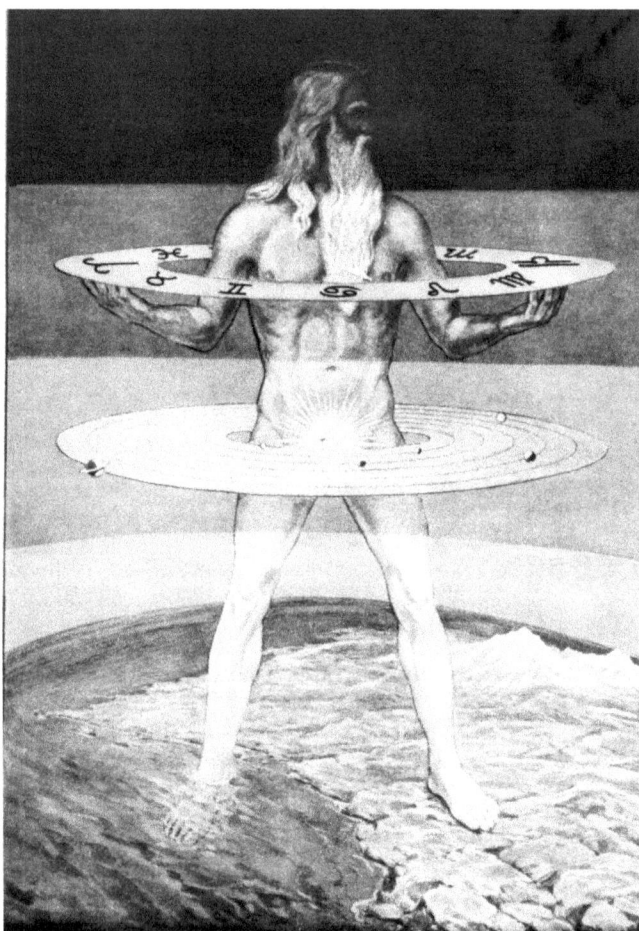

© Manley P. Hall

ORIGIN, HISTORY AND DEVELOPMENT OF LYMPHATIC MASSSAGE

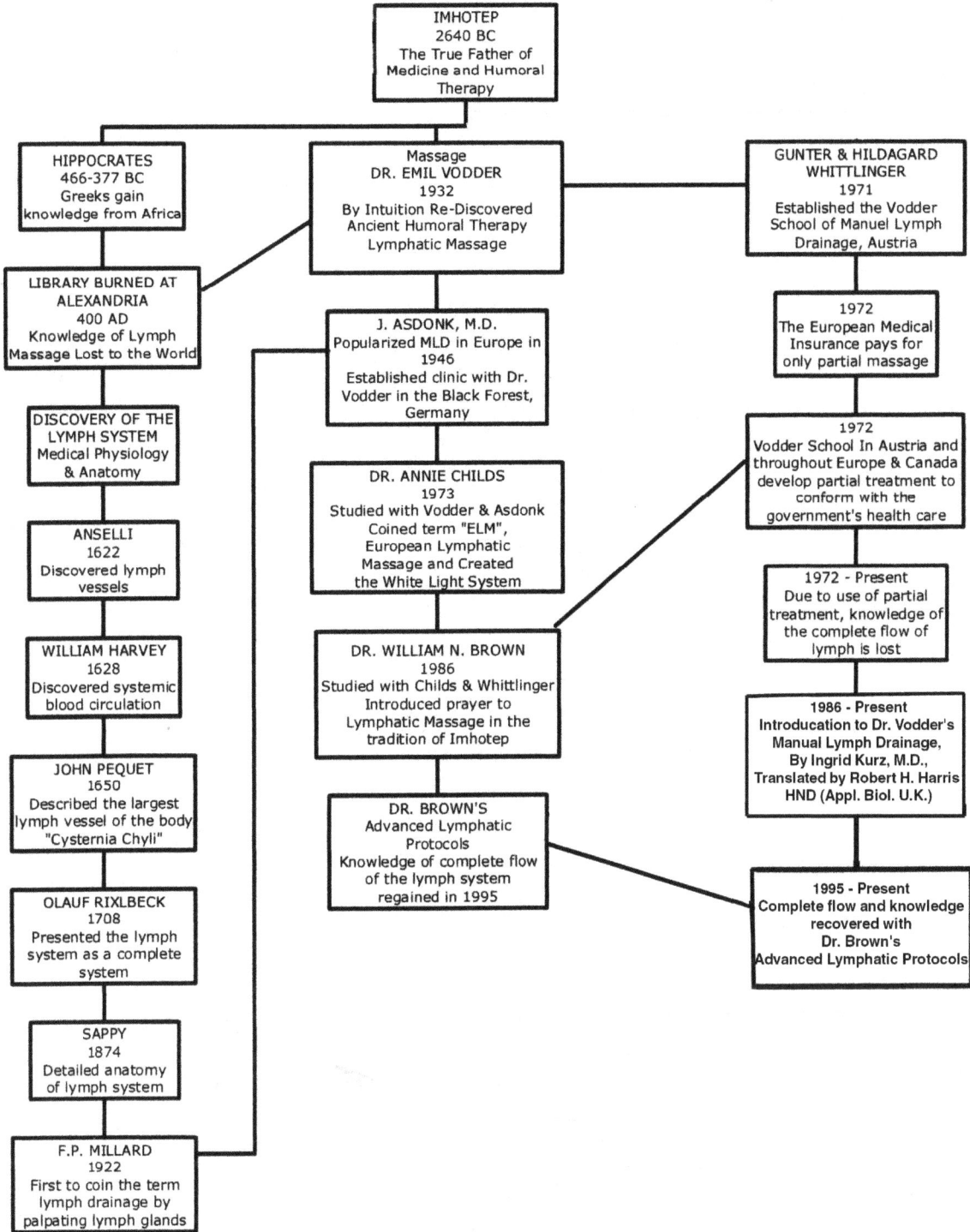

IMHOTEP
2640 BC
The True Father of
Medicine and Humoral
Therapy

HIPPOCRATES
466-377 BC
Greeks gain
knowledge from Africa

Massage
DR. EMIL VODDER
1932
By Intuition Re-Discovered
Ancient Humoral Therapy
Lymphatic Massage

GUNTER & HILDAGARD
WHITTLINGER
1971
Established the Vodder
School of Manuel Lymph
Drainage, Austria

LIBRARY BURNED AT
ALEXANDRIA
400 AD
Knowledge of Lymph
Massage Lost to the World

J. ASDONK, M.D.
Popularized MLD in Europe in
1946
Established clinic with Dr.
Vodder in the Black Forest,
Germany

1972
The European Medical
Insurance pays for
only partial massage

DISCOVERY OF THE
LYMPH SYSTEM
Medical Physiology
& Anatomy

DR. ANNIE CHILDS
1973
Studied with Vodder & Asdonk
Coined term "ELM",
European Lymphatic
Massage and Created
the White Light System

1972
Vodder School In Austria and
throughout Europe & Canada
develop partial treatment to
conform with the
government's health care

ANSELLI
1622
Discovered lymph
vessels

WILLIAM HARVEY
1628
Discovered systemic
blood circulation

DR. WILLIAM N. BROWN
1986
Studied with Childs & Whittlinger
Introduced prayer to
Lymphatic Massage in the
tradition of Imhotep

1972 - Present
Due to use of partial
treatment, knowledge of
the complete flow of
lymph is lost

JOHN PEQUET
1650
Described the largest
lymph vessel of the body
"Cysternia Chyli"

DR. BROWN'S
Advanced Lymphatic
Protocols
Knowledge of complete flow
of the lymph system
regained in 1995

1986 - Present
Introduction to Dr. Vodder's
Manual Lymph Drainage,
By Ingrid Kurz, M.D.,
Translated by Robert H. Harris
HND (Appl. Biol. U.K.)

OLAUF RIXLBECK
1708
Presented the lymph
system as a complete
system

1995 - Present
Complete flow and knowledge
recovered with
Dr. Brown's
Advanced Lymphatic Protocols

SAPPY
1874
Detailed anatomy
of lymph system

F.P. MILLARD
1922
First to coin the term
lymph drainage by
palpating lymph glands

Fig. 4

"I know that touching was and is and always will be the true revolution."

Nikki Giovanni

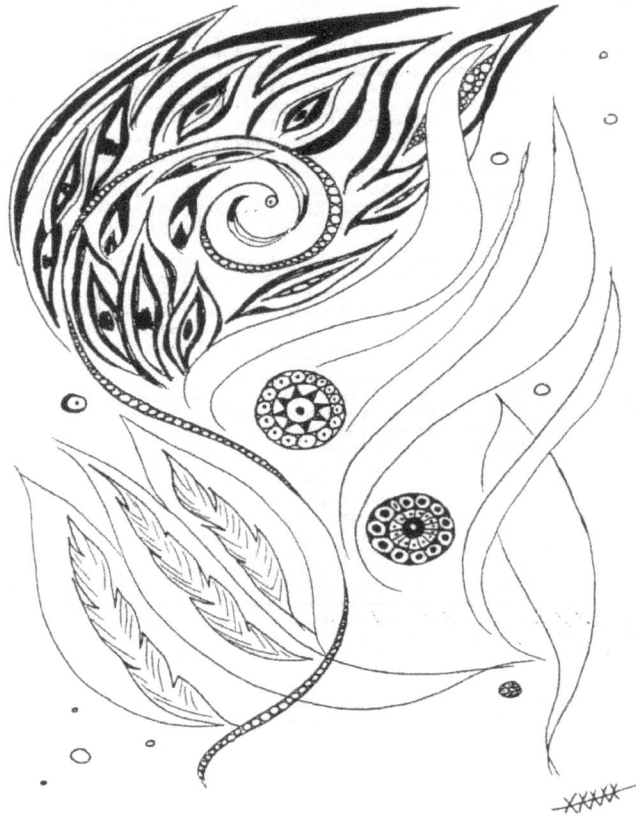

PART ONE

WHAT IS THE LYMPHATIC SYSTEM AND WHY IS IT SO IMPORTANT?

The lymphatic system nourishes the body by carrying nutrients to the cells. Lymph travels through channels that the circulatory system cannot reach. It is the cleansing, detoxifying, and rejuvenating system. It is our immune system. The lymphatic system produces white blood cells that attack invading bacteria and viruses while producing antibodies. It aids in the healing of problems associated with other systems of the body such as muscular, circulatory, respiratory, digestive, endocrine, nervous, and the elimination systems.

The most important problem is the disorders of the humeral system which are caused by these phenomena and the consequences which come from the behavior of individuals (IE. diet or lifestyle) in a normal or pathological state. The Hebrews and Egyptians, then later Hippo crates, already attributed the major part of morbid incidents to troubled humors.

By "humors" we mean the extra-cellular liquids of the organism. They form the fluid part of the circulating blood: the plasma, in which the sanguine elements appear, such as the suspended white and red cells, and also all the interstitial liquids either lacunal or others, which bathe, impregnate or encircle the tissue and organs. The "humors" may also be called lymphatic fluid. (Fig. 1)

The designation, lymph, was Bartholin's name for clear body water in 1652, and covers nutritive liquid on its way to cells, interstitial lymph as well as fluids within billions of cells (cytoplasm), which makes up half of the lymph fluid besides the lymph flowing through vessels and filtered by the lymph glands. The human body consists of 2/3 fluid, most of which is lymphatic fluid.

The lymphatic system in recent years has been a step-child of the medical profession. However in this century, the ancient humeral therapy is finding its place in modern healing practices. In recent years, an abundance of experience from clinical investigations and daily practice have brought about new discoveries of the structure and function of the lymphatic system. To quote Professor Cecil Drinker from a research work of Alexis Carrel, "the lymphatic system is the most important organic system of human and animal life; therefore we are now obliged to consider this system as one of the most important therapeutic factors in geriatric cases."

Lymphatic Massage is a massage technique developed in the 1930's by Dr. Emil Vodder, a European Physical Therapist. He called the ancient humeral art of lymph stream acceleration Manual Lymph Drainage and it is the most revolutionary therapeutic healing system to be rediscovered in the modern world. In the lymph stream, due to stress or some biological disturbance, certain inhibitors (mineral or organic) in the blood diminish in concentration. This is called the "soma tide cycle" by Dr. Gaston Naessens, and it continues its natural evolution and

Humoral Regulation of the Lymphatic System

"Humoral" refers to the fluid of the body, in other words, the extracellular fluid (ECF, which includes the blood plasma). For hormones whose secretion is regulated humorally, the endocrine cell responds to changes in the concentration of a substance in the ECF. The function of these hormones is the **homeostatic regulation** of the concentration of substances in the ECF. The hormones act to *stabilize and maintain* the concentration of the substance within the appropriate physiological range. Hence, the trigger for hormone secretion coupled to the hormone's actions in the body forms a **negative feedback loop**.

The figure schematizes humoral regulation of hormone secretion as a negative feedback regulatory system. Note that the endocrine cell acts as the sensor. The minus sign indicates that the action of the hormone is to oppose the disturbance that triggers its release. For example, an increase in blood glucose stimulates insulin secretion, and the effect that insulin has on its targets is to stimulate glucose uptake and utilization, and therefore to lower blood glucose.

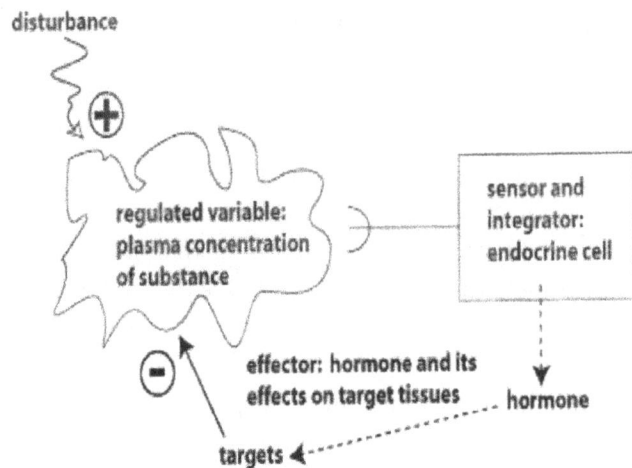

Fig. 1

one sees the appearance of diverse forms of bacteria in the body humors. These have also been termed Syphonospora Polymorpha, by German scientists during the 1930's.

With the technique of Lymphatic Massage, 40-50 liters of lymphatic fluid are accelerated, which results in the regulating of homeostatic disturbances of metabolism. All biochemical processes are only possible when the lymph flows through the cells. Accelerating the current of lymph flow allows a quicker detoxification process, and improvement in metabolism, and the betterment of conditions for life's processes.

Many difficulties for older people, and young too, could be avoided if it were understood that the lymphatic system is an all penetrating system, cleaning as well as rejuvenating. The joints will keep their strength and suppleness when regulating the synovial fluids through lymph drainage, because this process immediately starts the production of protective interferon. Every treatment is thus augmenting the body's own immunological forces. Your immune system is what protects you from the enemies around and within you such as bacteria, viruses, cancer, and atherosclerotic plaques. Without your immune system, you would have to live in a plastic bubble because the slightest exposure to bacteria or viruses will quickly lead to a deadly infection. As we age, our immune system's ability to protect us deteriorates seriously. In fact, most of us die because our immune system fails to protect us. Using lymphatic detoxification, nutrient supplementation and dietary modulation, we can dramatically improve the performance of our immune system, whatever our age.

The immune system is made up of the thymus gland and several types of white blood cells, which identify, attack, and eat deadly substances and produce substances like antibodies. The immune system also includes bone marrow, which makes some of the white blood cells; the spleen; the lymphatic system; nodes; ducts; capillaries; arteries; and a variety of protein and polypeptide weapons designed for the body's defense and repair.

The thymus gland is very important in the function of the immune system. However, after puberty this gland fails to function with the same efficiency. The thymus gland instructs certain white blood cells, called T-cells, as to what to attack and when. Without these instructions, these T-cells may fail to attack bacteria, viruses, and cancer.

Arthritis is believed to be a disease stemming from the attack of our own T-cells on our joint membranes and fluids. The T-cells create free radicals which are used in attacking enemies like bacteria, viruses, and cancer cells, but when the thymus malfunctions, T-cells can make mistakes and attack our own cells. In arthritis, the chemically reactive free radicals damage the joint membranes and lubricants.

Nutrients and modalities which improve the immune system's functioning can often provide dramatic relief of arthritis symptoms both by improving the ability of T-cells to differentiate self from other and by stopping the chain reactive damage of free radicals in the system.

As we grow older, we become less and less able to handle disease. The diseases of old age most likely to kill or disable us are arteriosclerosis, cancer, and arthritis. These can be prevented by a well functioning immune system. If you were able to maintain the physiological condition you had at early adulthood, you might reach a lifespan of over 800 years! The immune system is very important in determining your physiological condition.

What are the parts of your immune system? It consists of about one trillion lymphocytes and 100 million trillion antibody molecules, along with other chemical weapons such as interferon and tissue of bone marrow, spleen, thymus, and lymph nodes. As the red blood cell is the medium of transport of oxygen to the body, the lymphocyte is now proven to be a similar medium of transport for nucleic acids. It is important to note that it is the lymph that distributes all nourishment, mineral salts, vitamins, and oxygen from the blood to the cells. (See Fig. 2)

Many diseases are a result of cellular malnutrition due to lymphatic stagnation; eczema, chronic inflammation, traumatic edema, osteoporosis, allergies, and Hodgkin's disease, which was originally called lymphogranulomatosis.

Lymph drainage, when administered by specialists, is a natural, rational, cleansing of focal infections, especially is nasal, tonsillar, and dental affections. The latest research has proven the efficacy of this therapy.

Through these new special lymph drainage movements, dangerous, stagnating waste matter is eliminated. Accelerated production of lymphocytes is also achieved, which carried through the lymph and blood stream augment both immune defense and new building processes.

According to Dr. Arthur C. Guyton, Text Book of Medical Physiology, the removal of proteins from the interstitial spaces by the lymph system is an absolutely essential function, without which we would die in approximately 24 hours.

According to Dr. Gerald L. Lemole, Chief of the Department of Thoracic and Cardiovascular Surgery at the Deborah Heart and Lung Center, Brown Mills, New Jersey, the lymphatic system is not studied very much, most medical texts devote only one or two paragraphs to it, but the little known lymphatic system has three very important functions:

1. To return proteins to the blood.

2. To remove toxins and foreign particles. We are taught that the liver and kidneys carry away toxins, but it is actually the lymphatics that carry away the fluid that bathes each cell of our body.

3. As an integral part of our immune system.

According to Dr. Paschal M. Spagna, Chief of Cardiac Surgery at the Graduate Hospital, University of Pennsylvania, states lymphostasis or lymph stagnation is a critical factor in heart disease. He continues, the cardiac lymphatics are responsible for carrying away cholesterol from the intercellular spaces. If the lymphatics are blocked, the cholesterol cannot go anywhere, it stays in the walls of the arteries too long, thus contributing to arteriosclerosis. This idea is consistent with the

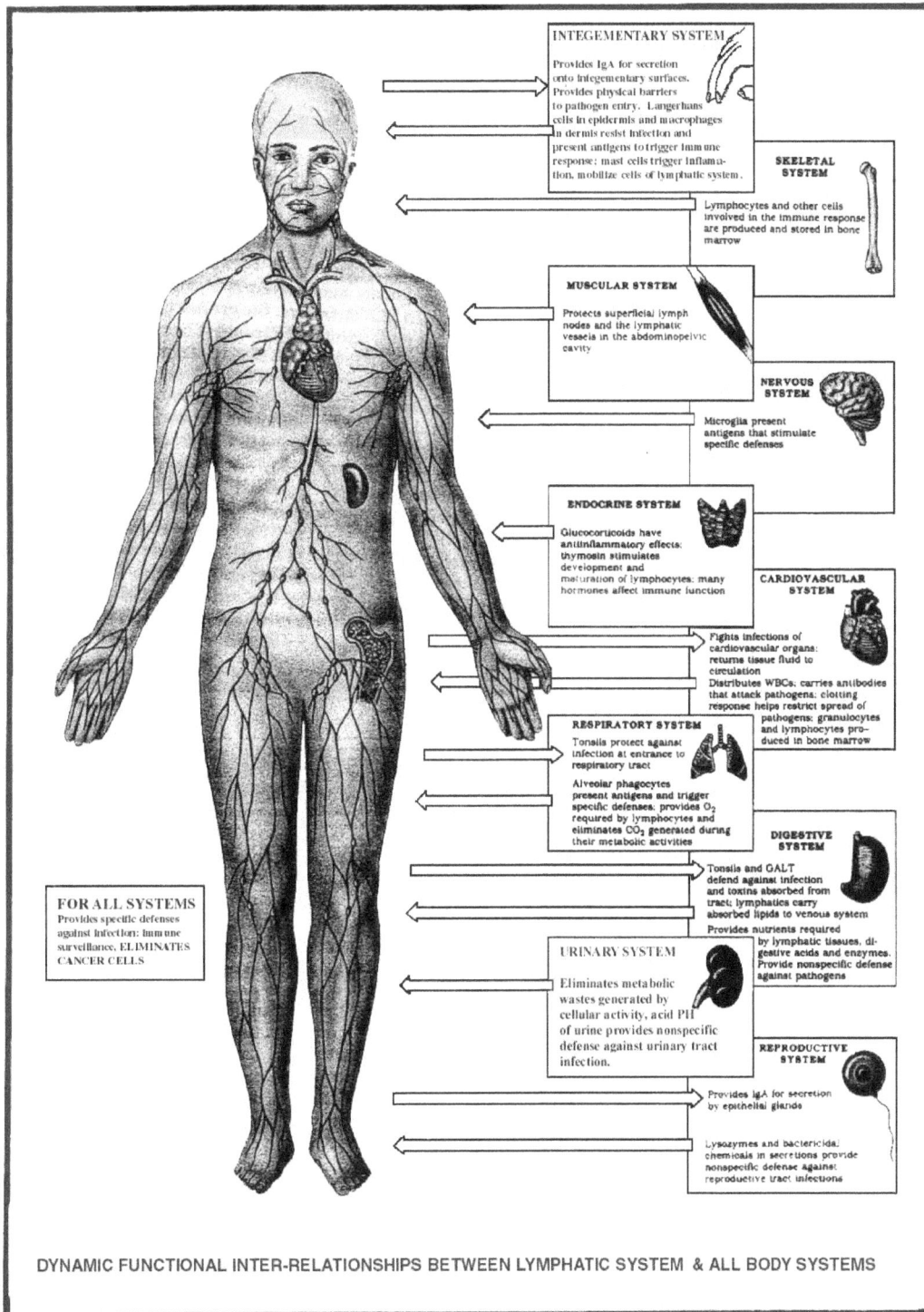

Fig. 2

fact that in 90% of the cases of coronary arteriosclerosis, postmortem examination shows scarring, inflammation, and blockage of the lymphatics.

In addition to heart disease, lymphostasis may be a contributing cause of cancer, because when the lymphatics are blocked, toxic molecules cannot be moved away from body cells and constant exposure to toxins may be a cause of malignancy.

"The main purpose of lymphatic drainage is to accelerate the movement of the lymph flow by partly emptying the tissues, an action not unlike clearing a stagnating pool. Just as important is the regenerating power of the drainage movements, an effect not to be found in the hard, inelastic massage technique." The renewing of tissue lymph makes possible the inflow of daily nutritional requirements and the building materials for regeneration and growth.

Thus, lymph drainage therapy supports the natural impulse of the body to purify and rebuild. Manual Lymph Drainage has been researched over the past twenty years by such scientists as M. Foldi, E. Kuhnki, and others. Its physiological benefits are well documented.

Lymphatic Massage is a precise technique designed to promote the normal functioning of the lymphatic system. The removal of metabolic wastes, excess water, toxins, bacterium, viruses, broken cells, plasma proteins, large fat molecules, and foreign substances from the tissues via the lymphatic vessels and venous capillaries is facilitated by Lymphatic Massage. Therapeutic application of Lymphatic Massage enhances the activity of the immune system, reduces pain, and stimulates the parasympathetic nervous system, which in turn alters the brain wave pattern to one which more closely resembles brain waves that are associated with the reduction of stress. Thus as a bio-energetic approach to massage, lymphatic massage therapy demonstrates benefits on the physical, emotional, and psychological levels of the human experience, with profound implications for enlightenment and transformation as an expression of God's love in elevating the entire planet to a higher octave of healing vibrations.

NUTRITION AND THE IMMUNE SYSTEM

Today more than ever, we are committed to our health. We take the time to eat right, exercise, and maintain positive mental attitudes. We do this all to stay healthy. After all, the benefits of being healthy are increased happiness and a longer life!

We eat right to provide the body with the necessary fuel for energy and rebuilding from the cells out. We exercise to strengthen and cleanse our body. We maintain positive mental attitudes which means releasing stress and worry, which can be major factors in illness.

The term nutrition comes from the Greek "*trophe*", which means to nourish. Trophology then is the study of nutrition. After the four major food groups (dairy, fruits, grains, and meats), I believe nutrition falls into some general categories:

1. QUALITY - such as unprocessed foods as opposed to highly processed and synthetic foods. Any kind of food processing is likely to change the nutritional value of foods and in many instances the quality of the food will be reduced. For this reason, we should use nutritional supplements.

2. PREPARATION - raw and steamed as opposed to fried foods. It has been shown in animals that the fat in fried foods leads to the death of cells, followed by a period of increased gas in the digestive tract. Obviously, diet can influence the potential toxicity to the cells.

3. COMBINATION - vegetables with proteins or vegetables with starches as opposed to proteins with starches or proteins with fruits. Food combining is very important. Our bodies cannot digest proteins and starches or proteins and fruits at the same time. The starches or fruits are digested first and the proteins last. For the body to work most efficiently, these foods should not be eaten at the same meal.

4. PSYCHOLOGICAL EFFECTS OF THE DIGESTIVE PROCESS - such as the state of mind when eating; angry as opposed to peaceful, hurried as opposed to leisurely. What you eat and how you eat affects how you feel. This observation is the result of a study on mood, carbohydrates, and obesity.

Scientific research has also shown that an improper diet is bad for your immune system. Undigested proteins in the blood stream are removed by white blood cells, which are a part of your immune system. Therefore, the immune system is being used for digestion rather than disease prevention. Also, the greater the intake of sugar, the lower the immune response.

It is important to remember that nutrition is not just food, but all that the senses encounter that feeds and nourishes the body. Scientific research has proven the need for nutritional supplements because of the processing of foods, environmental pollutants and toxins in the air and water, and our mental stresses. Thus it is important that we plan to use nutritional supplementation (vitamins, minerals etc.) in our daily diet. We have nutritional programs available to us which can assess our nutritional status and needs, and provide us with the nutritional insurance needed to maintain health and well-being in today's mechanical and industrial environment. Dr. Horwitt, in his interpretation of vitamin requirements stated that "Clinical evidence of Vitamin E deficiency was ameliorated by administration of Vitamin E in patients with malabsorption syndrome and in premature infants." Furthermore, to cure a Vitamin D deficiency in a patient, amounts of vitamins far larger than the daily requirement had to be used. This was necessary to speed recovery and replace deficient stores. Dr. Simopolus, states in agreement with Dr. Roger Williams, that variation in nutritional requirements and differences in genetic makeup suggest different vitamin requirements for different individuals. After years of nutrition research and practice, I can state categorically that dietary habits that are healthy strengthen the immune system. Clearly, health building programs are really immune strengthening programs!

Health programs using nutrition and physical medicine are not new. As far back as the 18th century, medical doctors used nonevasive therapies to treat disease. Notable among medical practitioners of this era was Dr. John Harvey Kellogg, founder of the health sanitarium in Battle Creek, Michigan. Dr. Kellogg treated his patients with nutrition, massage, and hydrotherapy (water therapy). He saw this as primary health care, and envisioned his health center as a model for the entire medical field. His dream faded with the advent of Allopathy (modern drug oriented medicine).

However, Dr. Kellogg's dream has been revived and appropriately utilized in what is now called preventative health care. Now, I do not believe that we can prevent the onset of old age or all the illness that may attend it, but I do believe that the symptoms of old age may be delayed and well-being maintained far into our twilight years. Preventative health care could be defined as immune strengthening through nutritional and dietary awareness, physical medicine or massage, psychological stress reduction and the acceptance of the responsibility for one's own health.

Massage of the skin holds a prominent position in alternative or preventative health care. The skin provides a barrier against disease by mechanical and chemical factors, and is an active part of the immune system. Dr. Ashley Montague in his book Touching, in the chapter titled "The Mind of the Skin" states; "We conclude, then, that the study of mammal, monkey, ape, and human behaviors clearly shows that touch is a basic behavioral need much as breathing is a basic physical need....and when that need for touch remains unsatisfied, abnormal behavior will result." Furthermore, Dr. Kellogg states in his book, The Art of Massage, relative to disorders of nutrition, "that ancient as well as modern physicians have regarded massage as a measure by which the general nutritive process of the body may be influenced to a powerful degree, by its effect on the circulatory system, the nervous system, and its effect on digestion, assimilation, and all the processes of secretion and excretion."

The human body is approximately 70% water. Balance is maintained in the body by fluid mechanics. There are protein buffers in the blood which maintain the pH of the blood. The blood pH must remain in very narrow pH limits of 7.35 to 7.45. However, in trauma, shock or stress, these blood proteins may leave the blood stream and enter the lymphatic system. These plasma proteins have to remain in the blood circulation. If there is a loss of proteins at a small rate of approximately 1/25 of the total proteins in circulation per hour and if these proteins are not returned to the blood circulation, death would ensue within 12 to 24 hours.

When we eat food, and digest it, the food is hydrolyzed which means it is broken down with enzymes in a fluid medium. The nutrients are absorbed into the blood stream, through the arteries to the arterioles, to the capillaries where the lymph leaves the blood stream carrying the nutrition to the cells. Bathing the cells with nutritive fluid, cleansing the cellular environment, and removing wastes and trapped proteins and returning them to the blood are all functions of the lymphatic system. Furthermore, the lymphatic system balances the hormones of the body, transports all the fat soluble vitamins which it picks up directly from the colon. In short, the lymphatic system runs through the whole body and is essential in rejuvenating the body. The lymphatic system is the immune system.

In the nucleus of the cell, the DNA and RNA are responsible for maintaining and replicating the genetic information in the cell. Scientists have noticed that changes in the environment of DNA (the cell) such as temperature, acidity, salt level, and water content, can change the DNA structures. This fact is very important, because the water in the cell is lymphatic fluid and can be affected by lymph stream acceleration.

Lymph stream acceleration or Lymphatic Massage is defined as: the process of quickening the vital waters and energies of the body with the resultant therapeutic benefits of cleansing, nourishing, and regenerating on a systemic (whole body) level. Lymphatic Massage is a dynamic, systemic, massage of the whole person, creating a unity of body humors (or fluids) and immune stimulation. Blood, sweat, tears, saliva, urine, mucus, cerebrospinal fluid, kyroplasm, cytoplasm, and digestive juices all develop from the embryonic sac of saline nutritive water and form the lymphatic system and lymph fluids. These fluids in the lymphatic system bring nutrition to the cells, and health and immunity to the whole body.

Wouldn't it be wonderful if we could just walk into our doctor's office and say, "I want you to increase my body's ability to use nutrients, balance my hormones, reduce my level of stress, cleanse my body, strengthen my immune system, and do it all in one hour!" Sound far fetched? Not at all, because all of this can be accomplished with Lymphatic Massage. This revolutionary technique is an immune strengthening gentle massage, developed in Europe in the 1930's by Dr. Emil Vodder of Denmark. Refinement of Lymphatic Massage by Dr. Asdonk, in a clinic in the Black Forest region of Germany, and research done by Foldi, Mislin, and others have proven the effectiveness of this technique. This modality is fully accepted by the medical insurance plans in Europe and doctors write prescriptions for this treatment on a routine basis there. (This technique was refined and improved by Dr. Vodder's student, Dr. Anita Childs.) I studied Lymphatic Massage with Dr. Childs, and have practiced it for over 25 years with excellent results. These results are even greater when combined with holistic nutritional therapy.

Holistic nutrition deals with the scientific, intuitive and metaphysical aspects of nutrition. When we eat in a healthy, harmonious way, our ability to attune and commune with the Divine is enhanced. With this idea, I suggest that rather than "living to eat" or "eating to live", that we eat to increase our ability to be in communion with God. I believe that diet should completely support the spiritual life of any person within any religious or spiritual path.

For proper nutrition to be of maximum benefit, it should be integrated into a harmonious balance of right life, good fellowship, wisdom, meditation, prayer and love. It must be realized that food is a dynamic force which interacts within the body on the physical level, within the mind and emotions, and also on the energetic and spiritual level. Therefore the art of Holistic nutrition is the application and understanding of the interaction with and the assimilation of the energetic aspects of food by the creative forces of the total being; mind, body, and spirit.

ELECTROMAGNETIC ASPECTS OF FOOD AND LYMPHATIC MASSAGE

Milk cyclone fermentation can have D-positive or D-negative aspects in the living cell. It has been proven that the prolonged left turning cycle of D-negative milk ferment is a cause of cell deterioration, stopping cell respiration and causing the cells nucleus to form cancer. Dr. Engelhardt demonstrated that the heart muscle can only use D-positive milk cyclone for its electrochemical balance and strength.[1]

There are many other muscles that require the same maintenance and repair. The organ of the skin is particularly influenced by D-positive foods. D-positive milk cyclone activates the lymphatic system and helps to detoxify the entire body from environmental and other poisons. Lymphatic massage, therefore, is what we can do to improve our immune system. With lymphatic massage, wounds heal faster (including ulcers of the leg), swollen glands start to decrease as the tissue becomes better nourished and the accumulated waste is expelled.

The lymphatic fluid is under the influence and affected by the magnetic field. Many women may gain three to five pounds of fluid when the moon is full and may loose that amount two to three days later. Many hyperactive people become super-hyper when the moon is at it's peak of shining. Doctors may recommend sedatives are used twice as much for hyper-active children under the influence of the moon.

We have not paid enough attention to the electromagnetic influence of the environment on our lymphatic system. Lymphatic massage will ease many woes in a simple and multifaceted and holistic way. Your life is in the blood because the lymph is in it. And it becomes the light of electromagnetic knowledge.

The secret power behind the movement of the lymph is magnetic in nature. The movement of each individual blood cell, the joining together, the giving up of energy to each other, the lumping together as blood clots; behind all this is electromagnetic power, the secret of the universe, the untapped energies of the cosmos working in our lymphatic system.

With lymphatic massage, the hands are directed by the will and are instruments which will correct a faulty magnetic life pattern in the lymphatic stream. This massage will influence and strengthen a faulty electromagnetic pattern.

---

[1]   Kroger, Hanna, God Helps Those Who Help Themselves

THE 5 DEBILITATING INFLUENCES WHICH CREATE AN OPPORTUNITY FOR THE MANIFESTATION OF ELECTROMAGNETIC IMBALANCE

1. Stress

2. Diet

3. Emotions

4. Thoughts

5. Environment

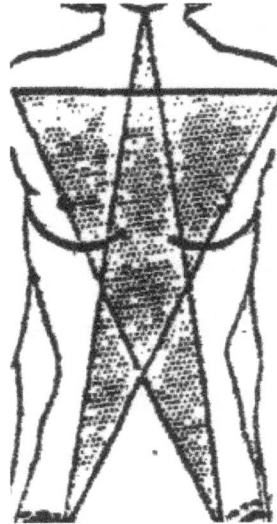

Research has proven that water can be structured and re-structured with emotion outside the body[2]. Lymphatic Massage can re-structure the water inside the body utilizing exactly the same principals. It is the structure of the water in the body (lymph) and the relationship to the emotions (love) that indicate health. The electromagnetic current in the body (vitality) is increased with lymphatic massage which also balances all the systems of the body by harmonizing the frequency or vibration of the lymphatic system to the emotional frequency of love.

---

[2]   See Dr. Emoto's work on the emotion's effect on water.

FOODS & HERBS THAT SUPPORT THE LYMPHATIC SYSTEM

1. Coffee - Indian and New Guinea. Good for spleen support of the immune system and lymph.

2. Beets/Carrots - helps cleanse and support the lymph

3. Amino Acids - help strengthen the immune system

4. De Cystothionion -

5. DL Hydroxylysin

6. DL Norvalin

7. Herbs for the spleen - chaparell, cayenne, golden seal, echinacea

8. Red clover Burdock root

9. Chlorophyl

10. Ligustrum

11. Clevers

12. Poke root

13. Mullein

14. Lobelia

NUTRITION TO CLEANSE AND SUPPORT THE LYMPHATIC SYSTEM

1. **Lymph Congestion**

Start with 5 juniper berries a day. Chew them slowly between meals twice daily. Every day add 1 juniper berry so you'll have 6 juniper berries twice daily. Increase to 15 juniper berries twice daily. Then, every day, reduce the number to 1 berry until you are on the statu ratio 5 twice daily. By chewing, take one by one. Since there are 15 berries, it will take you close to one hour to chew so many.

Congestion in the lymph system is most favorably influenced by this method.

2. **Lymph Cleanser**

Barley: Boil three tablespoons barley in one quart water for thirty minutes. Add a little clove and cinnamon. Drink this in one day, it will clear the congestion in the lymphatic system.

Applewhey:

Take one pint apple juice or apple wine.
One pint water
One pint milk

Heat slowly, but do not bring it to a boil. When it curdles, strain it through a fine cloth, throw curds away, sweeten with honey, if needed. Take two tablespoons five times daily if person is very weak. Appetite will come soon. As patient gets stronger, give up to two cups a day, it is powerful.

3. **Decongest your Lymphatic System**

1 pint white grapefruit juice
1 pint freshly squeezed orange juice
1 pint grape juice
1 pint water with the juice of three limes
1 pint water with the juice of two lemons
1 pint frozen pineapple juice, diluted
1 pint papaya juice, diluted
12 eggs (whole)
6 egg yolks
frozen raspberries or strawberries add a delicious flavor

Beat eggs and mix into fruit juice mixture.

This is a one day's supply. If you are hungry, add one kind of fresh fruit. For lunch, green salad and/or sprouts with raw almond dressing. For supper, green salad and/or sprouts with almond dressing and one steamed vegetable.

4.   **Lymphatic System Cleanser**

Cucumber: Four to five cups a day for a week of cucumber juice purifies the lymphatic system and the blood and clears the complexion.

Recipes for lymphatic cleansing provided by Hanna Kroeger, *God helps those that help themselves*, 1984. Rev. Hanna Kroeger.

When you kill animals for food, you disrupt the electromagnetic balance of the cells in the food.. If you eat living food, it will strengthen you, but if you kill your food, the dead food will kill you also. Life only comes from life, and death always comes from death. Everything which kills your food kills your bodies also, and that which kills your bodies kills your souls.

Truly we must view the body as the temple of the living God and food as our offering to the divine spirit that lives in the body temple. When we speak of Holistic nutrition, then prayer and meditation are the spiritual food which feed us on the royal road to the attainment of inner freedom. It is the sustenance which allows us to reach from earth to heaven, from weakness to strength, from darkness to light. There is a power and energy in our food which gives strength not only to our bodies, but also to our hearts, minds, and spirits. The source of this strength is not the food, the individual body or mind, but rather that aspect deep inside each person that knows the truth!

MANUAL LYMPH DRAINAGE

Manual Lymph Drainage is a massage technique. It is an ancient technique rediscovered in the 1930's by Dr. Emil Vodder, a European physical therapist. MLD has been researched over the last 20 years by such scientists as, Professor Foldi, Professor Mislin, Dr. Asdonk, and others. It's physiological benefits are well documented, however, its psychological benefits are just recently being explored. In various countries in Europe, Manual Lymph Drainage is covered by government health plans and is therefore prescribed by physicians and practiced in hospitals for many medical problems. Unfortunately, to meet government requirements for national health plans, the technique has been changed from full body therapy to a piecemeal approach. <u>See. Fig. 3, Pg, 22.</u>

Manual Lymph Drainage is a precise and intricate technique designed to promote the normal functioning of the lymphatic system, by accelerating the flow of the lymph stream. It is used primarily in the treatment of edematous tissue and various chronic inflammatory conditions. Manual Lymph Drainage facilitates the removal of trapped plasma proteins, metabolic wastes, excess water, toxins, bacteria, viruses, dead and broken cells, large fat molecules and foreign substances from the tissue via the lymphatic system. Therapeutic application of Manual Lymph Drainage enhances the activity of the immune system, reduces pain, and stimulates the parasympathetic nervous system. Manual Lymph Drainage is a very gentle process with a very profound effect.

It can be generally said that there are four major effects of Manual Lymph Drainage on the body. These are:

1. The effect on the autonomic nervous system, including its effect on the reflex pathways.

2. The immunological effect.

3. The effect on the smooth muscles of the blood and lymph vessels.

4. The drainage effect.

The autonomic nervous system consists of the sympathetic nervous system, or the awake or conscious system, which makes us active and allows us to work, and the parasympathetic system, the sleeping or unconscious system, which permits us to rest, and renew our strength. These two nerve systems extend to all parts of the body, vessels, muscles, organs, the skin and even branch out into the soft connective tissue.

In a healthy person, the autonomic nervous system is balanced. Daily stress, diet, the environment, and striving for success are factors which contribute to the fact that many of us no longer possess a balanced autonomic system. As a result, the sympathetic nervous system predominates, thereby decreasing our ability to relax.

Manual Lymph Drainage has a stimulating effect on the parasympathetic nervous system. This means that after proper application of the technique the client becomes calmer, more relaxed. Some even fall asleep during the treatment. This effect is desirable, there are a number of clients whose disease stems from the fact that they are in a state of disharmony in which the sympathetic system dominates their body.

It is therefore essential that the Manual Lymph Drainage techniques be carried out in a gentle, slow, precise rhythm. If performed too quickly, they will have just the opposite effect. The parasympathetic system has a trophotropic effect; that is, it promotes growth and recovery and restores strength. These are processes that are characteristic of sleep and cannot be influenced by conscious will. The causes of muscular hypertension are often of a subconscious nature. In using Manual Lymph Drainage, we are able to influence muscular hypertension through the parasympathetic nervous system.

While the conscious mind in man is centered in the cerebrum, the sources of unconscious nonphysical stimuli are assumed to be seated in the autonomic centers of the rest of the brain and the spinal column. Reflexes that can be triggered by physical massage act upon these autonomic centers.

Dr. Vodder's lymph drainage is based on an ingeniously devised, simple and effective technique that brings about an acceleration of lymph flow. At the same time, a soothing effect on the sensitive nerve endings of the skin is achieved.

A reflex is a response to a stimulus. Nerve cells called receptors are organs designed to receive various kinds of stimulus. There are receptors that respond to light, chemical substances, heat, and mechanical influences. The various types of stimulus result in different reflexes. Many reflexes are accompanied by feelings. The reflexes that are of interest to us are the "fight or flight" reflexes, as well as those that induce pleasure. Hard, rough massaging may set off recoil and defense reactions or even flight reflexes. The resulting pain is usually associated with increased muscle tension. Feelings of aversion (such as anger, fear) accompany these reflexes, and are indicative of the somatopsychic relationship of body and mind.

However, when Manual Lymph Drainage is properly employed, pleasure reflexes are elicited. These are accompanied by pleasant sensations (such as feelings of affection, well being). They lower the basic activity of the muscles and thus exert a relaxing effect.

The nerves known as nociceptive fibers transmit pain-causing stimuli from the periphery in the form of electrical impulse to the spinal column and thence to the brain. The nociceptor continues to send impulses or more technically, action potential, to the central nervous system as long as it is excited; that is, as long as the cause of the pain persists.

Besides nociceptors, there are also touch or pleasure receptors. These transmit stimuli produced by touch, such as those that are elicited by Manual Lymph Drainage or stroking. The pleasure receptors transmit touch sensations by means of action potential via nerves to the spinal column. There, through a complex series of interactions with the transmission of the nociceptor stimuli, the receptors establish an inhibitory synapse (which means that any pain signals coming from the nociceptors are inhibited, blocked, even canceled),whenever the inhibitory cell is simultaneously excited. There is, however, one exception. The touch receptor responds to changes in the stimulus, for example, at the beginning and at the end of a stroke, but not to the stroke itself. Therefore, it is continuously excited by Manual Lymph Drainage, and since the constantly changing pressure applied during Manual Lymph Drainage brings along a continuous variation in stimulation. The touch receptors and the inhibitory cells are continuously excited.

This means that precise execution of Manual Lymph Drainage, which is characterized by light, continually changing pressure, activates inhibitory cells whose function is to decrease or even eliminate sensations of pain.

The immune system distinguishes between "self" and "other". In the body the feature "self" is carried to a large extent by proteins, but also polysaccharides and neurohormones. In the larger molecules of multicellular animals, certain chemical groups possess a spatial arrangement that is characteristic of the species. This species-specific spatial pattern within the molecule is the genetically coded self feature, or DNA. It is by virtue of this special molecular arrangement that every living species claims its uniqueness. It is the function of the immune system to protect this uniqueness, and maintain its viability.

The immune system is directed not only against infectious pathogens, but also against substances that are foreign to the species, especially proteins. Pathogens (bacteria and viruses) that possess virulence, antigenicity, or both will trigger the defense mechanisms of the immune system. However, due to the psychosomatic aspect of the mind body relationship, the immune system will also respond to negative thoughts.

In addition, the immune system is responsible for getting rid of body tissue that has no function, as this represents a disturbing influence in the protein individuality of the organism (IE. the removal of pre-cancerous cells via the lymph stream).

The immune system constitutes a vital protective system of the body. Immunity is understood to be the protection we have against a second attack of an infectious disease.

Two mechanisms are responsible for immunity. Firstly, proteins (globulins) are the vehicles of the defense function. These are called antibodies and are the mediators of humoral immunity. Secondly, there are cells (lymphocytes, plasma cells, phagocytes, macrophages) that can render detrimental substances harmless. This is called cellular immunity.

The immunological benefit of Manual Lymph Drainage resides in the fact that pathogenic substances present in the body fluids are transported rapidly by manual massage to the lymph nodes, where they are inactivated. Generally speaking, successful defense against infection by microorganisms depends on the degree of resistance and the presence of immunity. Resistance is understood to be the entire defense complex that the body can mobilize against the antigens of a pathogen before the immunological response is initiated. Resistance is not antigen-specific. It is determined by genetic and environmental factors (nutrition, exhaustion, disease). There is no doubt that resistance is strengthened by regular Manual Lymph Drainage.

We also know through observation that Manual Lymph Drainage influences immunological events and that the treatment of mucous membranes with Manual Lymph Drainage yields good results. This is because the habitat of IgA antibodies is maintained or even improved.

Manual Lymph Drainage has a tonic effect on the smooth muscles of the blood vessels, it causes the precapillary sphincters (the closure muscles at the beginning of a capillary) to contract. This is evident during Manual Lymph Drainage by the fact that the skin pales. Once the sphincters close, the capillary pressure drops. This increases the edema-reducing, resorptive capacity of the capillaries, resulting in drainage of the tissues.

The lymph vessels are constructed differently from the blood vessels. The lymph vessels are built up of individual valve segments, called lymphangiones. Each of these lymphatic segments has a valve that opens in only one direction. This determines the direction of lymph flow and prevents backflow. The ring-shaped smooth muscles of the segments contract in response to various stimuli and press the contents of the lymph vessels, the lymph, in the direction in which the valves open.

Stimulation of various nerves leads to contraction of the lymph vessels, either actively or reactively. Therefore, the lymph volume in the peripheral lymph vessels determines the pulsation rate and thus the transport rate of the lymph. Stimuli are produced by:

      a. Movements of the skeletal muscles

      b. Pulsation of the arteries

      c. Movement of the diaphragm during breathing

      d. Peristaltic movements of the intestine

      e. The pressure differences which occur during respiration

The major influence on pulsation, however, comes from stimuli evoked by stretching, either from inside, i.e. during filling of the vessel lumen, or from outside. An example would be by gentle displacements of the skin as practiced in the special lymph drainage technique developed by Dr. Vodder.

When vessels contract actively, as the lymph vessels do, the vessels then play an important part in fluid transport, as in lymph drainage massage. A closer look at lymph drainage massage reveals that there are three types:

1. Extravascular lymph drainage involves lymph formation and extravascular circulation. Lymph is formed from blood plasma which finds its way into the interstitial spaces by filtration or diffusion, from various proteins, which enter the

interstitial spaces in the same manner and/or by active transport (cytopempsis), from large-molecular fat molecules from the digestive tract, and from non-migratory cells.

The more protein there is in the tissue, the less water can flow out of the tissue via the venous blood capillaries, because protein retains the water. By transporting protein out of the interstitial spaces, the lymph system again permits more water to flow out through the blood capillaries.

2. Extramural lymph drainage, i.e. the external mechanical effects on the lymph vessel, is based on the fact that the external forces not only stimulate the vasomotor system, as described above, but also act mechanically on the contents of the lymph vessels. Among these external forces are the movements of the skeletal muscles, the pulsation of the arteries, the peristaltic motion of the intestine, the movements of the diaphragm and the other respiratory muscles, and the pressure differences which arise alternatingly in the thoracic and abdominal cavities during breathing.

3. Auxiliary, indirect lymph drainage, which is supported locally or regionally by manual, direct lymph drainage massage.

The unique massages of Manual Lymph Drainage stimulate the lymphatic motor system. Physiologic vasomotor lymph drainage is based on the autonomic pulsations of the chain of lymph sections. Manual Lymph Drainage exerts a decisive influence on this system of drainage. The process is achieved by the rhythmically repeating of the Manual Lymph Drainage techniques, causing a peristaltic wave of contractions. Also, stretching stimuli increase the "pulse rate" of the lymph sections. Smooth muscle cells, such as those in the vessel wall, exhibit electrical and mechanical reactions after undergoing passive stretching. To regulate their stimulation, the vessel wall muscles require a measured stretching which is dependent on the degree to which the vessels are filled. Manual Lymph Drainage, imparts a tensile (stretching) stimuli and thereby brings about a stimulation of vasomotor lymph drainage. In addition, increased lymph production, as through Manual Lymph Drainage, can also lead to more rapid lymph drainage.

When we speak of drainage in connection with Manual Lymph Drainage, we are referring to the removal of fluid from soft connective tissue. Thus we transport water and substances from loose connective tissue via the lymph system. These substances are referred to as the lymph-obligatory load. Water is also removed via the blood vessel system, after the water holding plasma proteins are removed by the lymph system.

The treating of the lymphatic system is not simple, because lymph vessels are of fragile structure, as thin as silk threads, and the capillaries are still more delicate. The classic massage movements have no real draining effect: hard, inelastic pressure also empties the deeper blood vessels, thus preventing new regenerating plasma from flowing into the tissue. A painful destruction of vessels and capillaries is often the result, seen as hematomas. Therefore Manual Lymph Drainage is a useful new technique.

In order to obtain a water pumping effect, we have elaborated movements going in and out of tissues. When such refined circular spirals are used, with consciousness concentrated in the fingertips, like the touch of a cat's paw, a perfect relaxation of tissue is obtained. This condition allows new lymph to penetrate, with pure oxygen and fresh building materials, regenerating all organs and tissues. The patients experience a real rejuvenation.

Dr. Asdonk took part in a one-month course in Copenhagen, and later, established a clinic in the Black Forest Region of Germany where he taught Manual Lymph Drainage with Dr. Vodder. He described the drainage movements in the following way: "These delicate circular massage movements, going into tissue with oblique spirals in many variations, are following the mechanical laws for flowing water with such a high degree of accuracy, that a maximum of water distribution in tissues is obtained, together with a perfect outflow through the lymph vessels. It is a well elaborated massage method."

In nature, all life's unfolding movements, turn in spirals; here in our drainage, moving in and out of tissue, rhythmically, crescendo - decrescendo, in the same way as the heart beats, pumping during the systole, relaxing during diastole. The cycle of the heart last eight-tenths of a second, and rests four-tenths of a second; the heart works exactly as long a time as it relaxes. Therefore, the heart is able to live and work a hundred years without getting tired. This important pause of the heart is called by the French: "Le grand silence du coeur", by the Germans: "Die schopferische Paulse", it means: the creative pause! All physiotherapists that learn lymph drainage massage should also study Tai-Chi Chuan so they can work non-stop without being tired and exhausted. When working relaxed and harmoniously, one feels nature's sources flowing. They could be called cosmic forces.

Tai-Chi is an ancient art that embodies the three principles of: 1.Yin-Yang, which may be described as a blending of opposites; 2. meridians that are said to contain a free flowing colorless noncellular liquid, and are described as energy pathways traveling throughout the body linking organs and body parts; and 3. Chi which is vital energy or life force. Chi flows through the meridians providing essential energy to the organs and body. Chi is necessary to the existence of life. The principles found in the philosophy of Chinese medicine of which Tai-Chi is an integral part, reveal a deeper insight to the nature of lymphatics and an intuitive acknowledgment of spirit. Alexis Correl reached the same conclusion thousands of years later when he demonstrated with his experiment in the 18th century that organs could not sustain life in the absence of lymph flow. Chinese medicine views the body as a whole, consistent with the admonition of Dr. Vodder that the technique of Manual Lymph Drainage be performed as a full body therapy. The Nei Ching (the ancient Chinese medical manual on acupuncture) states in its description on the flow of Chi through the meridians to the organs of the body, that the function of the Yin organs is to produce, transform, regulate and store the fundamental substances.

Chi is divided into the four fundamental substances of blood, Jing, Shen (defined as spirit), and body fluid. Jing is described as essence and called the substance that underlies all organic life and the source of change. This essence is described as a fluid which is supportive, nutritive, and is the basis of reproduction and development. Clearly, this is lymphatic fluid. The only fluid that exists at the interstitial tissue level or the intracellular level is lymphatic fluid. The concept of Chi is not well understood in the West, nor the acceptance of meridians, but somehow acupuncture still seems to work. Could we be overlooking the lymphatic system again? Could the undetectable energy meridian system be the lymphatic system? It would appear so.

Acupuncture balances the internal flow by the use of needles which control the emptying or filling of vessels and organs with Chi which is carried in the lymphatic fluid. Manual Lymph Drainage balances the internal flow by the acceleration of the lymph stream which empties and fills the vessels and organs with lymph fluid, in which the Chi is carried, to bring balance to the entire system. Both acupuncture and Manual Lymph Drainage work on the same system, however Manual Lymph Drainage is less invasive.

The lymphatic system is the immune system which forms the basis of healing in all methods, particularly Manual Lymph Drainage. The ancient description of the nature of lymphatic fluid has profound implications regarding the emotional, energetic and spiritual aspects of Manual Lymph Drainage. The highest form of healing occurs when science, philosophy, and religion merge in recognition of spirit. Manuel lymph drainage, however, in its present form, still practiced in stages which interrupt the accelerated flow of the lymph. (See Fig. 3) Advanced Lymphatic Protocols facilitate the incorporation of the complete flow of the lymphatic system. I hope to see this lymph drainage massage method introduced everywhere in the world. The medical profession and its helpers may use it as an effective auxiliary therapy, and suffering mankind will benefit by an intensive, nurturing method of treatment.

M.L.D. SEQUENCE
Emmaline Barker, M.S.T., M.L.D.

Neck

Arms   When you have finished the 3 week treatments you have given three

Chest   full massages.

Abdomen   2 ½ treatments = 1 whole

Legs   18 full treatments should cleanse the whole lymph system in a
                            <u>healthy normal person</u>..

Nape

Back

loins

WEEKLY TREATMENTS

1st Week   2nd Week   3rd Week   (First week repeat 2nd & 3rd weeks)

1st Day	2nd Day	3rd Day	4th Day	5th Day
Neck	Neck	Neck	Neck	Neck
Arms	Abdomen	Nape	Abdomen	Nape
Chest	Legs	Back	Loins	Face

TWO ONE-HALF DAYS PER WEEK

1 - One-Half Treatment   2 - One-Half Treatment

Neck	Neck
Arms & Chest	Abdomen
Abdomen	Nape
Legs	Back
Face	Loins

Fig. 3

LYMPHATIC MASSAGE
THE QUICK, EASY, SYSTEMIC APPROACH
TO MANUAL LYMPH DRAINAGE

Manual Lymph Drainage is a connective tissue massage technique originated by Dr. Emil Vodder of Denmark in the 1920's. More specifically, Dr. Vodder said that he was intuitively led to do this gentle, circular, healing with his hands. It is clear, according to Dr. Vodder's own words, that he channeled this ancient knowledge. In fact Dr. Gutman, in referring to Dr. Vodder's work, said that it was part of the ancient humoral therapy. After exhaustive research of world history, particularly of old Greece and Nubian Egypt, it has been determined that humoral therapy was practiced by Imhotep, a Nubian priest/ healer/architect of the step pyramids in Central Africa. Later, he created a healing pyramid temple at Heliopolis on the banks of the Nile. There he practiced humoral therapy by accelerating the vital humors of the body (lymphatic fluid) and utilizing gem stone color therapy as a complete form of vibrational and energetic body healing. The Greeks, who were the progenitors of western civilization, gained their knowledge of medicine philosophy, science and mathematics from Black Africa or more specifically from Nubian Egypt. The Greeks held this knowledge gained from Africa in high esteem and referred to one of their major teachers, Imhotep in the Hypocratic oath as Aesculapius. Imhotep has been called the true father of medicine by Dr. Charles Drew, the creative medical pioneer and inventor of the technique of blood transfusion.

This ancient knowledge of humoral therapy was lost when the library at Alexandria, Egypt was burned in 900 A.D. It can be said that the knowledge of this work was maintained in the universal collective unconscious of mankind, and was intuitively rediscovered by Dr. Vodder in the late 1920's. Together with Dr. Jonas Asdunk, Dr. Vodder developed and taught the technique in Denmark, Germany and France, which was called European Manual Lymph Drainage.

From Vodder's work, two major schools of technique have developed. The traditionally structured school of Manual Lymph Drainage in Germany teaches Dr. Vodder's official technique. The European school of lymph drainage is a highly structured institution, teaching basic through advanced therapy. The American school's greatest proponent has been Dr. Vodder's student, Dr. Annie Childs. Dr. Childs, through her medical background and over forty years as a massage therapist (competent in all major existing modalities), has created a Neo-Vodderian approach to Manual Lymph Drainage. She has termed this technique the Lymphatic Massage and it is taught in a less formal structure than the European school. The American system consists of a three part seminar series encompassing; basic, advanced and special treatments which include cellulite control. The seminar graduates form a network of practitioners from coast to coast and throughout the United States.

Due to the common origin of these two approaches to lymphatic therapy, Manual Lymph Drainage and Lymphatic Massage, there are many similarities. There are however, some very important differences. Differences which as massage therapists, we need to grasp and understand in order to propitiously utilize these techniques to help our patients. The first basic difference between the European school and its American counterpart would be the consideration of time. The European school, because of its traditional approach requires a greater financial and time commitment in order to complete the courses, some of which can only be completed in Germany. The Neo-Vodderian approach of Dr. Childs provides a therapist with a systemic and skillful technique which can be readily applied with efficacious results in a very short period of time. This ease of application is facilitated by the creative genius of Dr. Childs' approach to teaching and by the dynamic structure of the technique of Lymphatic Massage as she recreated it. Manual Lymph Drainage is a precise and specific technique which is difficult to master. It requires a great deal of precision and practice. As applied through the technique of Lymphatic Massage, it is no less precise, yet the improvements and refinements Dr. Childs has created, allow the application to be easier while the effective therapeutic results remain extremely consistent.

There are many questions that could be examined concerning the distinction of one technique as opposed to the other. A few of the more important differences between Manual Lymph Drainage and Lymphatic Massage are: Manual Lymph Drainage is mechanistic, clinical and divided into parts, while Lymphatic Massage is bio-energetic, intuitive, and systemic. With Lymphatic Massage, a full body massage takes between 45 minutes and one hour, in Manual Lymph Drainage, full body is between 1½ and 2 hours. The bio-energetic aspect of Lymphatic Massage (i.e. the massage and control of energy flow) makes the technique different in concept and application. Differences may also be determined by patient need and the structure of your practice. However, the philosophic differences between Manual Lymph Drainage and Lymphatic Massage may affect your approach to the therapy. The differences in philosophy are more than the result of differences of personality between students of the same teacher, but rather a result of years of experience and knowledge of massage combined with intuitive spiritual direction and innovation on Dr. Childs' part to adapt European Manual Lymph Drainage to the American lifestyle. The result, the Lymphatic Massage, is not only consistent with, but can enhance the American lifestyle. This quick and easy approach strengthens the immune system and eliminates stress, which makes it perfect for the American fast paced, high stress way of life.

The fact that there are at least two major interpretations of therapeutic application of lymph drainage, and other less effective methods (Ayurvedic and Chiropractic approaches to lymph drainage to name but a few), gives therapists a wider range of opportunity and choice in the development of their skills in the art of lymphatic massage.

The essence of the art of Lymphatic massage is that it is easy, gentle and forgiving. It is an intuitive skill that can be acquired quickly. The technique of Lymphatic Massage combines Tai-Chi, Yoga, creative visualization, intentionality, and multi-dimensional evolutionary experience with the healing touch! The healing touch is what triggers the immune system to respond at a higher frequency like love, Agape, Bakti which are devotions of the heart.

Lymphatic Massage allows the practitioner to function in a space of self development, humility and spirituality. The healing of self, love of God, and work in the light are the principles on which Lymphatic Massage are based. With Lymphatic Massage one may experience the tenderness of the Earth Mother and the compassion of the Universal Father, allowing an energetic healing to be coaxed through the heart and hands to strengthen and rejuvenate the entire immune system. Lymphatic Massage is one of the highest and finest spiritual arts I have ever known. I am honored to practice and privileged to teach this ancient system of healing.

The technique of Lymphatic Massage is easy to learn, the cost is reasonable, three day seminars are $750.00. The philosophic approach to the bio-energetic application of Lymphatic Massage benefits both the therapist and patients with renewed energy and vitality. While Manual Lymph Drainage is an excellent physical therapy, Lymphatic Massage is the only technique that requires the practitioner to say a prayer before beginning the work. The practitioner then must remain in a prayerful, meditative state throughout the application of the treatment. This higher state of mind during the procedure of Lymphatic Massage is what moves it beyond physical therapy into a multi-faceted Holistic approach to energetic mind, body, and spiritual balance.

The protocols for European Lymphatic Massage are very different from MLD. In lymph massage we recommend ten (10) treaments with three (3) within 24-48 hours, the remaining seven (7) can be done on a weekly basis. These ten treatments were established by Dr. Vodder and Dr. Johanas Asdonk. They determined that dequbitis ulcers could be cured with ten (10) lymphatic whole body treatments. The piecemeal approach used in MLD is not consistent with the intent of Vodder, nor does it facilitate an effective complete flow of the lymphatic system. It is a technique of parts where the sequence of parts do not equal the whole or greater than. However lymphatic massage is a technique of wholism, a systemic approach whereby the whole is greater than the sum because it includes spirit.

I must conclude from my experience under the expert tutelage of instructors from both disciplines, that what is most important is that this very powerful, subtle, and therapeutic modality be seen by the world in its true light as part of the healing of the living waters of this planet. That it be made available to those therapists who are and will be the light bearers to facilitate the movement of the healing waters of life as an expression of God's love and light in transforming and healing the planet.

LYMPHATIC MASSAGE,
A NATURAL HELP FOR THE IMMUNE COMPROMISED INDIVIDUAL

Lymphatic Massage, the art and science of lymph stream acceleration, may hold the greatest possibility of increasing the quality of life for individuals suffering from immune system dysfunction. The lymphatic system is a virtually unknown circulatory system related to the cardio-vascular system, which is part of it and separate from it at the same time. It is our immune system. To understand the immune system, we must first start at the cell, the building block of the body.

The cell is composed of three basic parts:

1. The cell wall, more technically called the phospholipid membrane, which serves as a gatekeeper. It allows fluid into the cell carrying nutrients and out of the cell carrying wastes.

2. The cytoplasm inside the cell wall which serves as a energy factory with various components suspended in this fluid media.

3. The nucleus which contains the DNA helix and serves as the command center.

It is important to note that in all three aspects of the cell, it is energized, supported and maintained in a fluid medium. That fluid is lymphatic fluid, the river of life which maintains balance (IE. health) in the internal environment. In fact, the fluid in the nucleus is called karyolymph and is key to the health, structure, and replication of the cell.

It has been discovered that what drives the structure of the DNA helix inside the nucleus of the cell is temperature, pressure, and hydration. The significance of this discovery has a profound effect on how we view our approach to manual medicine and the healing of the human body, based on cell replication, rejuvenation, and homeostatic equilibrium. The fluid inside the nucleus of the cell when in proper balance, creates an ideal environment for the correct replication of new cells. However, an imbalance of fluid may create the production of faulty cells and in turn, cellular degeneration. It is important to know that the fluid in the nucleus of the cell is the same fluid that runs in tiny vessels under the skin, called lymphatic vessels. Therefore the balance of the fluid on the inside of the nucleus of the cell can be influenced merely by touching the skin in a spiral, rhythmic, wave-like motion.

The lymphatic fluid carries nutrients to the cells, cleans the cellular spaces (both internally and externally) and also maintains the life force through homeostatic equilibrium. The function of the immune system is to protect us from outside invaders and internal renegade cells, which divide and proliferate out of control (IE. cancer cells). The exogenous invaders may include, but are not limited to: germs, viruses, bacteria, fungi, worms, parasites, processed foods, synthetic chemicals, smoke, venoms, etc. Anytime these substances enter the body, they trigger an immune response. The immune system first identifies the invader, then acts to destroy it. The foreign invader is called an antigen. White blood cells carried in the lymphatic stream call macrophages, consume the antigen. Then the macrophages signal other white blood cells called T-cell lymphocytes, which in turn release substances called lymphokines. The lymphokines stimulate other white blood cells called B-cells to make antibodies. Antibodies are chemical proteins that adhere to antigens and cause them to be attacked and devoured by other scavenger white bloods carried in the lymph stream, called phagocytes. Through the technique of Lymphatic Massage, the lymph stream is accelerated carrying the phagocytized antigens, toxins, cancer cells etc. away to be excreted by the organs of elimination (liver, kidneys, bowels).

In the case of immune system disfunction, specifically the HIV virus, it is in the nucleus of the T-4 cell that the virus integrates itself in strands of the DNA helix. Within the nucleus of the cell, the HIV virus uses a protein enzyme called reverse-transcriptase to insert itself on to the DNA chromosomes. This allows the virus to act as a gene and become a template of information which takes over the production function of the DNA itself. This causes new virus genes to be made which kill the host cell and go in search of other lymphocyte cells to infect. Literally millions of lymphocyte cells are produced in the bone marrow every few minutes. Infected individuals must strategically strengthen their immune system with natural therapies and Lymphatic Massage, which demonstratively strengthens and tones the immune system. This will knock out the viral invaders before they can progress too far. Of course, good nutrition is paramount to a strong and healthy immune system.

In ARC(AIDS related complex)/AIDS patients, the immune system becomes compromised due to a number of mind/body/spirit factors. As a result of this lack of strong immunity, germs which we all carry within our bodies at all time, get the opportunity to multiply unchecked.

The list of germs, bacteria, fungi, viruses, and antigens that affect ARC/AIDS patients grows longer each day. The following are just a few:

> Pneumocystis Carinii
> Candida Albicans
> Herpes Simplex
> Epstein-Barr
> Viruses (HIV, etc.)

Recently there have been correlations made between AIDS and Chronic Fatigue Syndrome. In the past, Chronic Fatigue Syndrome was thought to be a form of depression. The neurohormone serotonin in the brain, alleviates depression. Since Lymphatic Massage increases this neurohormone, its impact on Chronic Fatigue Syndrome would be obvious.

However, in 1992 researchers identified cases of AIDS without HIV infection. The non-HIV AIDS cases had many similar syndromes that exist in HIV AIDS cases, IE the destruction of T4 cells resulting in suppressed immunities. Further research has demonstrated that many non-HIV AIDS cases were really Chronic Fatigue Syndrome.

In both AIDS and Chronic Fatigue Syndrome immunodeficiencies include not only the destruction of the T4 cells, but also the inhibition or incapability of natural killer cells of the immune system. These natural killer cells are one of the most important aspects of the body's defense against virus and infectious bacteria. It has been shown time and again by many different practitioners, that the symptomology of Chronic Fatigue Syndrome can be modulated systemically with as little as 10 treatments of the Lymphatic Massage.

Also, cancer is common in immune compromised individuals. There is evidence to suggest that there may be common universal determinants in the development of cancer. Electromagnetic pollution, synthetic chemicals, vitamin and mineral deficiencies, viral particulates, and negative mental attitudes. All seem to have involvement in a comprehensive theory concerning the cause of cancer. The one single element that ties them all together is a compromised immune system.

Here are a few alternative theories as to the causes and prevention of AIDS and AIDS related syndrom:

WHAT REALLY CAUSES AIDS: An Executive Summary

By: Harold D. Foster

The AIDS pandemic is likely to become the greatest catastrophe in human history. Unless a safe, effective vaccine is quickly developed, or the preventive strategies outlined in this book are widely applied, by 2015 one sixth of the world's population will be infected by HIV-1 and some 240 million people will have died from AIDS. Its associated losses by then will be more than those of the Black Death and World War II combined, the equivalent of eight World War Is. [1]

This pandemic is only one of several ongoing catastrophes involving viruses that encode the selenoenzyme glutathione peroxidase. [2] *Indeed, the world is experiencing simultaneous pandemics caused by Hepatitis B and C viruses, Coxsackie B virus and HIV-1 and HIV-2. As these viruses replicate, because their genetic codes include a gene that is virtually identical to that of the human enzyme gluthathione peroxiase, they rob their hosts of selenium. Paradoxically, however, they diffuse most easily in populations that the very selenium deficient,* [3] *possibly because their members have depressed immune systems. It is no concidence that such viruses are causing havoc at the beginning of the 21ˢᵗ century. The last 50 years have seen enormous expansions in the use of fossil fuels and deforestation by fire. The resulting pollutants have greatly increased the acidity of global precipitation, reducing selenium's ability to enter the food chain. This situation is being made worse by the widespread use of commercial fertilizers since their sulphates, nitrogen, and phosphorus all depress the uptake of selenium by crops. Deficiencies in this essential trace element are being felt most acutely in areas, such as sub-Saharan Africa, where soil selenium levels are naturally very low. Acid rain is making a bad situation worse, so increasing vulnerability to those viruses that encode glutathoine peroxidase. Many populations are also being exposed to a thinning ozone layer, heavy metals such as mercury and cadmium, pesticides, and drug, tobacco, and alcohol abuse , all of which depress the human immune system, increasing vulnerability to viruses, including HIV-1 and HIV-2.*

In July 2000, physicians and scientists from around the world met in Durban, South Africa for the XIII International AIDS Conference. In a declaration, named after the city, 5,018 of them proclaimed that, "HIV is the sole cause of AIDS."[4] There are, however, at least seven anomalies that strongly suggest that this conventional wisdom is incorrect and that belief in it is blocking progress in the development of new treatments for AIDS and of novel ways of preventing its spread. To illustrate, despite widespread unprotected promiscuous sexual activity in Senegal, HIV-1 is diffusing very slowly, if at all, amongst the Senegalese.[5] It is very apparent that in Africa, differences in soil selenium levels are greatly influencing who becomes infected with HIV-1 and who does not. Indeed, the recently published Selenium World Atlas used the incidence of HIV-1 as a surrogate measure of soil selenium levels because actual levels are, as yet, poorly established in sub-Saharan Africa. A similar relationship has been documented in the United States[6] where there has been an inverse relationship, especially in the Black population, between mortality from AIDS and local selenium levels.

It is well established that individuals who are HIV-positive gradually become more and more selenium deficient.[7] This decline, which is known to undermine immune functions, is not unique to HIV-infection but is seen in almost all infectious pathogens.[8] However, under normal circumstances, where death does not occur, selenium levels rebound soon after recovery. HIV-1, however, can effectively elude the defense mechanisms of the immune system, and can continue to replicate indefinitely, endlessly depressing serum selenium. As a result, the immune system is compromised, allowing infection by other pathogens that continue to deplete the host of selenium, allowing HIV-1 to replicate more easily, further undermining immunity. Therefore, this relationship between selenium and the immune system is one of positive feedback, in which a decline in either of these two variables causes further depression in the other. Termed the "selenium-CD4 T cell tailspin" by the author,[9] it is the reason that serum selenium levels are a better predictor of AIDS mortality than CD4 T cell counts. Like other positive feedback systems, such as avalanches and forest fires, it is extremely difficult to control and gains momentum as it progresses.

HIV-1, however, encodes the entire selenoenzyme, glutathione peroxidase. As it replicates, therefore, it depletes its host not only of selenium but also of the other three components of this enzyme: namely, cysteine, glutamine, and tryptophan.[10] AIDS, therefore, is a nutritional deficiency illness caused by a virus. Its victims suffer from extreme deficiencies of all four of these nutrients which are responsible for such symptoms as depressed CD4T lymphocyte count, vulnerability to cancers (including Kaposi's sarcoma), depression, psoriasis, diarrhea, muscle wasting, and dementia. Associated infections cause their own unique symptoms and increased risk of death.

HIV-A alone, therefore, does not cause AIDS. It involves a multiplicity of co-factors, specifically anything that either depletes serum selenium levels or depresses the immune system enough to permit viral replication. Manipulating the "selenium-CD4T cell tailspin" by adding this trace element to fertilizers and food stuffs opens new avenues for both prevention and treatment. This strategy has been shown to work on other viruses that encode glutathione peroxidase, such as Hepatitis B and C and the Coxsackievirus. The logical treatment of AIDS patients involves supplementation with selenium, cysteine, glutamine, and tryptophan, and Vitamin C at least to levels at which deficiency symptoms associated with a lack of these 5 major nutrients disappear. While this can be most easily achieved by supplements, certain foods contain elevated levels of those five nutrients, of which selenium is the highest.

References

1.   *Foster, H.D. (1976). Assessing disaster magnitude: A social science approach. The* Professional Geogapher, *xxviii(3), 241-247.*

2.   *Taylor, E.W. (1997). Selenium and viral diseases: Facts and hypotheses.* Journal of Orthomolecular Medicine, *12 (4), 227-239.*

3.   *Ibid.*

4.   *The Durban Declaration (2000),* Nature, *406, 15-16.*

5.   UNAID/WHO Epidemiological Fact Sheet on HIV/AIDS and sexually transmitted infections: Senegal. *2000 update (revised).*

6.   *Cowgill, U.M. (1997). The distribution of selenium and mortality owing to acquired immune deficiency syndrome in the continental United States,* Biological Trace Element Research, *56, 43-61.*

7.   *Baum, M.K., Shor-Posner, G., Lai S., Zhang, G., Lai H., Fletcher, M.A., Sauberlich, H., and Page, J.B. (1997). High risk of HIV-related mortality is associated with selenium deficiency.* Journal of Acquired Immune Deficiency Syndromes and Human Retrovirology, *15(5), 370-374.*

8. *Sammalkorpi, K., Valtonen, V., Alfthan, G., Aro, A., and Huttenun, J (1988). Serum selenium in acute infections.* Infection, *16(4), 222-224.*

9. *Foster, H.D., (2000). Aids and the "selenium-CD4T cell tailspin": The geography of a pandemic.* Townsend Letter for Doctors and Patients, *2009, 94-99.*

10. *Mariorino, M., Aumann, K.D., Brigelius-Flohe, R., and Doria, D.,van den Heuvel, J., McCarthy, J.E.G., Roveri, A., Ursini, F., and Flohe, L. (1998). Probing the presumed catalytic triad of a selenium-containing perdoxidase by mutational anaylsis.* Z. Ernahrungswiss, *37(Supplement 1), 118-121.*

Entire article available through the Author, Harold D. Foster, Department of Geography, University of Victoria, PO Box 3050, Victoria, B.C., V8R 6H3, Email: fhoster@coastnet.com.)

Was it an "accident" or "act of nature," that after HIV had curiously devastated two minority populations by 1995 – African (mainly female heterosexual) Blacks and gay American males – by 2000, the epidemic had shifted to strike mainly herterosexual Blacks and Hispanics in America?

Death in the Air

Fig. 14.2. Dr. Horowitz's Response to Dr. Satcher

NEWS RELEASE

Release: No. 97-EV/9
Date Mailed: June 18, 1997
For Immediate Release

CDC Director Pulls Invitation to Discuss Controversial Book on AIDS-linked Vaccines

Rockport, MA — Centers for Disease Control and Prevention (CDC) Director David Satcher, challenged by scientists, Black leaders, and citizen groups concerned about vaccination risks, declined to discuss AIDS as a possible outcome of contaminated vaccines with the author of a new and highly controversial book that documents the CDC and Food and Drug Administration (FDA) helped manufacture a vaccine that might have transmitted AIDS worldwide. The exchange between the author of *Emerging Viruses: AIDS and Ebola—Nature, Accident or Intentional?* (Tetrahedron Publishing Group, 1997), Dr. Leonard Horowitz, a Harvard graduate, independent investigator, and internationally known public health authority, and Dr. Satcher, followed a recommendation for a moratorium on vaccines by the Nation of Islam's Health Minister, Dr. Alim Muhammad, and a special legislative committee meeting of the National Medical Association, representing Black physicians of America, in which the book's main thesis, and supportive documentation, was considered. All parties agreed that growing fears over vaccine contaminations, and associated health risks, should be addressed at another meeting proposed, then cancelled, by Dr. Satcher.

Dr. Horowitz, supported by thousands of concerned citizens in a rapidly growing grass roots coalition, accepted Dr. Satcher's invitation in writing contingent upon an official investigation into the role the CDC played in "developing the vaccine that most plausibly delivered AIDS to the world." In his book, two man-made theories of AIDS's origin are advanced and bolstered by astonishing government documents including National Cancer Institute reports showing how much U. S. taxpayers spent for contracts to develop and test immune system destroying viruses on monkeys and humans. According to Dr. Horowitz's theory, the CDC, FDA, and Merck & Company, a leading vaccine manufacturer, developed 200,000 human doses of a potentially contaminated experimental hepatitis B vaccine that was given to thousands of Central Africans, gay men in New York City, and mentally retarded children on Staten Island, simultaneously in 1974—perfect timing for the initial outbreak of AIDS cases in these areas by 1978.

Fig. 14.2. Dr. Horowitz's Response Continued

In an official letter to Dr. Horowitz in which he withdrew his invitation to meet, Dr. Satcher stated the "CDC believes that scientific evidence is the foundation for sound public health policies," and that Dr. Horowitz's allegations "do not appear to be based on credible, evidence-based information."

In response, Dr. Horowitz reported to thousands of Internet-workers, and the press, that Dr. Satcher's comments were false and misleading. "If the CDC truly demanded rigorous scientific proof to support its public health policies," Dr. Horowitz said, then the CDC would also be calling for a moratorium on virtually all vaccinations "which, to date, lack definitive scientific analyses showing positive risk/benefit ratios." In fact, Dr. Horowitz wrote Dr. Satcher, CDC and pharmaceutical company experts "don't really know whether vaccines are harming or killing more people than they are helping or saving."

Likewise, Dr. Horowitz questioned how much scientific evidence the CDC and FDA officials demanded when their "mutual consent was given to blood and pharmaceutical interests to sustain the use of HIV contaminated clotting factor VIII and blood supplies to the public between 1983 and 1986," despite the fact that these officials predicted thousands would die as a result. Furthermore, in 1984, when the hepatitis B vaccine link to the AIDS epidemic was first advanced then investigated by CDC and Merck, Sharp & Dohme collaborators, homosexual men in New York City were known to be the primary and earliest test subjects for the suspected vaccine. Yet the CDC omitted the New York City gay men from their investigation and focused only on Denver and San Francisco populations that had not been immunized using the earliest, most implicated, vaccine lots. "No wonder your 'expert' CDC authors remained 'Anonymous' on this *Morbidity & Mortality Weekly Report*," Dr. Horowitz chided. "I too would feel ashamed to affix my name to such bogus 'science.'"

Taken from: ***Death in the Air: Globalism, Terrorism & Toxic Warfare***
Copyright, 2001
Leonard G. Horowitz, D.M.D., M.A., M.P.H.
Tetrahedron Publishing Group

THE FIVE INFECTIOUS DISEASES

1. *Bacterial*

2. *Virus*

3. *Staph*   ***THERE ARE 5 MAJOR KINDS OF
                     INFECTIOUS DISEASES, ALL OF WHICH
                     ATTACK THE BODY THROUGH THE***

4. *Virod*   ***LYMPHATIC SYSTEM*** (See Fig. 4)

5. *Fungus*

THE FIVE DEBILITATING INFLUENCES AFFECTING THE IMMUNE SYSTEM

1. *STRESS*

2. *DIET*

3. *THOUGHTS*   ***THERE ARE 5 MAJOR KINDS OF
                        DEBILITATING INFLUENCES, ALL OF
                        WHICH LEAD TO LYMPHATIC***

4. *EMOTIONS*   ***CONGESTION AND IMMUNOLOGICAL
                        COMPROMISE OR DISEASE***

5. *ENVIRONMENT*

Fig. 4 Immunological Affects of The Five Infectious Diseases

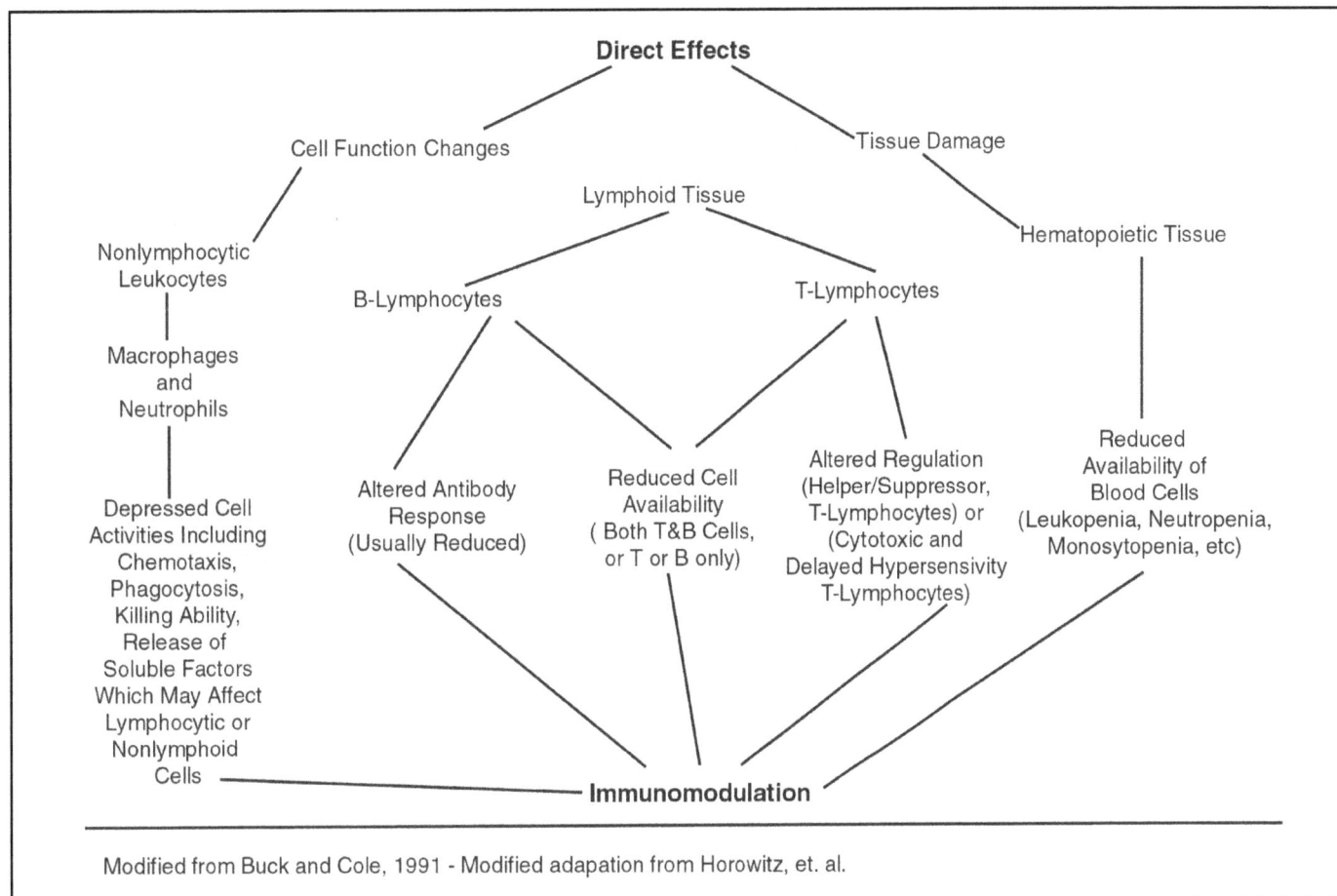

Direct Effects

Cell Function Changes — Tissue Damage

Lymphoid Tissue

Nonlymphocytic Leukocytes

Hematopoietic Tissue

B-Lymphocytes — T-Lymphocytes

Macrophages and Neutrophils

Depressed Cell Activities Including Chemotaxis, Phagocytosis, Killing Ability, Release of Soluble Factors Which May Affect Lymphocytic or Nonlymphoid Cells

Altered Antibody Response (Usually Reduced)

Reduced Cell Availability (Both T&B Cells, or T or B only)

Altered Regulation (Helper/Suppressor, T-Lymphocytes) or (Cytotoxic and Delayed Hypersensivity T-Lymphocytes)

Reduced Availability of Blood Cells (Leukopenia, Neutropenia, Monosytopenia, etc)

Immunomodulation

Modified from Buck and Cole, 1991 - Modified adapation from Horowitz, et. al.

With a strong immune system, the pentacular diseases, nor the pentagram of debilitating influences, can harm us. Through the application of regular lymphatic massage we can strengthen our immune system.

The five major benefits of lymphatic massage are:

1. Decrease stress;
2. Increase nutrient assimilation;
3. Release negative emotions;
4. Cleanse the internal environment; and
5. Normalize cellular function and repair tissue damage.

We know that germs and cancer cells are always present in the body. Only a strong immune system can hold these ever present enemies in check. Exactly how the immune system may fight various viruses may be infinite in its complexity. However, with the art of Lymphatic Massage, it can be reduced to the simplicity of gentle, precise and loving touch that eliminates stress and tones and strengthens the immune system. To this end, may the world know and use this heart-centered method that heals mind, body, and spirit.

Our immune system can be weakened by too little sleep, too much smoking, too much alcohol, by chemicals and pesticides, by metallic poisons (protoplasmic poison), by ELF Wave and others. Once your immune system fails to protect you, you are in trouble. Bacteria, virus, and fungus find a possibility to enter your blood stream, your lymphatic system, your cells.

Infections, diseases can be harmless or very serious. We are surrounded by bacteria, by fungi, by virus causing diseases, we are surrounded by protozoa, by all kinds of diseases. Those diseases cannot harm us as long as our immune system is fit.

With regular lymphatic massage, you keep your immune system strong and fit. A one hour lymphatic massage is equal to eight hours of sleep resulting in energetic and physical rejuvenation.

The beneficial effect of lymphatic massage on the immune system has been demonstrated over years of experiences. Lymphatic massage stimulates both specific immunological defense system and non specific immunological defense system, both cellular and humoral. This includes the antigen antibody reaction, the production of interferon, and the five different gamma globulins: (Ig A, D, E, G, M.). It is IGE which plays a prominent role in allergenic reactions and is released during the antigen antibody reaction.

LYMPHATIC MASSAGE,
THE TOUCH THAT HEALS THE THOUGHTS THAT KILL

There is evidence of a close interaction between the mind and the immune system. The scientific study is called Psychoneuroimmunology. One of the greatest proponents of this new science being Dr. Bernie Segal, M.D. This new science proves that man's mental and emotional nature affects his physical health. To gain a clearer picture of how this mind/body connection works, it can be explained that the mind and emotions work through the brain to start a chain reaction of hormone messages which are carried in the lymphatic stream. The lymphatic system is the immune system and is regulated by hormones secreted by the endocrine glands.

To gain a better insight to the function of the immune system, we can scrutinized the structure of the brain. Cognitive functions take place in the cortex, and are connected to the limbic system. It is in the limbic system of the brain that emotions are experienced. Both the limbic system and the cortex are connected to the hypothalamus which is located at the base of the brain.

It is in the hypothalamus that thoughts and emotions are integrated with the nervous system of the body. Mechanisms within the hypothalamus regulate the automatic functions of the body, IE. temperature, heart rate, and most important to immune system function, glandular secretions.

At the base of the hypothalamus is the master gland of the body, the pituitary gland. This gland is divided into two sections, anterior and posterior, and is half nerve and half gland. It is the hypothalamus that stimulates the pituitary to secrete its hormones. These hormones regulate other glands, including the thymus (which may be called the heart of the lymphatic system), and the adrenals and white blood cells (which are carried in the lymph stream). This entire system of brain, nerves, glands, hormones and white blood cells are structured in a circular feed back loop to interact and create balance through the entire system. This is how the mind and emotions in the brain, the hypothalamus and pituitary affect the immune system.

There are vast amounts of scientific documentation that prove bereavement, loneliness, lack of self esteem, and negative attitudes (such as hate, anger, and fear) depress the immune system. In many cases, the doctor's prognosis that a disease syndrome has no known cure, feeds the limbic system in a negative manner. The doctor's prophesies become a self-fulfilling body program for death. Clearly what we think affects how we feel and has a direct effect on our immunities.

We must realize that our minds can be used as a tool for our healing. We can choose to use it however we wish. We need not succumb to negative thought patterns. We can choose not to suffer, we can choose to be healthy and whole in our minds, bodies, and spirits.

As human beings, we act, feel and subsequently perform in accordance with what we imagine to be true about ourselves and our environment, both internal and external. The human brain and nervous system are engineered to react automatically and appropriately to the problems and challenges of life. We act, feel, and see, not according to what is really true, but according to the image our minds hold. We act as though this is reality, rather than our idea of reality. It follows, that if our ideas and mental images concerning ourselves are distorted or limited, then our reactions to our problems will also be distorted and inappropriate.

Our physical body has a built in thermostat, called homeostasis, which maintains our inner physical environment regardless of the extremes of the external environment. We also have a built-in spiritual thermostat which enables us to maintain an emotional/psychic atmosphere in spite of the emotional and psychic verities or extremes which may exist around us. Many people do not use their spiritual thermostat because they are unaware of it. They do not understand that they do not have to take on the outward climate or accept the pronouncements of so-called experts as truth. We can create our own reality, our own truth!

Our spiritual thermostat is just as necessary for emotional/psychic health and well being as our physical thermostat is for our physical health. Our mind, body, and spirit is and should be united with one purpose, one goal: health, wholeness, and glory to God. We cannot believe ourselves, "made in the image of God" deeply and sincerely, and not receive a new source of strength and power but we must choose to believe first.

The Lymphatic Massage facilitates this choice in a multifaceted way. First, it helps to alleviate stress which frees us of the psychological pressure of negative thought patterns. Secondly, Lymphatic Massage changes the neurohormones in the brain that cause depression and thereby elevating one's mood. Thirdly, Lymphatic Massage balances the endocrine system and the hormonal secretions through the body. This provides physical, emotional, psychological and therefore, spiritual balance throughout the entire being. Last, but not least, Lymphatic Massage provides for increased immunity, both specific and nonspecific, by cleansing and toning the entire immune system.

Lymphatic Massage is a heart centered, nurturing, gentle technique that through its very application allows for acceptance, support and intimacy in a nonsexual, nonthreatening way. Truly Lymphatic Massage is the touch that heals the thoughts that kill. May this spiritual art of Lymphatic Massage help to change the collective mass consciousness of the world, from death and destruction to one of love and light and life.

SPIRITUAL EVOLUTION THROUGH THE IMMUNE SYSTEM

Lymphatic Massage accelerates the lymph flow, quickening the elimination of toxins and harmful deposits in the tissues. Stress and overwork are conditions which cause the blood and lymph to stagnate. The metabolism of the cells becomes insufficient creating acid which poisons the environment of our tissues. This acidosis may cause pain, tension, and emotional imbalance. The Lymphatic Massage is beneficial because it releases stress, enhances the immune system and stimulates the nervous system to reduce pain.

In Europe, doctors prescribe Manual Lymph Drainage and it is practiced in hospitals. Europeans have benefitted from this technique for over 50 years. We can now demonstrate the fruit of the long development of this work in the refined technique of Lymphatic Massage.

The lymphatic system nourishes the body by carrying nutrients to the cells. It is also the system that cleanses and rejuvenates. Lymph travels through the channels of the body that the circulatory system cannot reach. Our immune system, with its complex hormones, white blood cells, prostaglandins, fat soluble vitamins, minerals, proteins and lymph fluid is part and parcel of our lymphatic system. A clean and balanced immune system may be the straightest and clearest path to enlightenment. When one is at peace mentally, which Lymphatic Massage facilitates through the reduction of stress, and when one is balanced physically (IE. hormonally) we have the opportunity to evolve to a profoundly deeper understanding of self. Evolution may be viewed as movement from one level to a higher level, with each succeeding level bringing one closer to ultimate source.

Disease manifests in the body when the lymphatic system becomes congested. This, therefore, blocks the energetic flow to our mind and distances our communion with spirit. Assuring that the lymph glands and vessels are healthy and free of congestion would probably be the best approach to preventing disease in mind, body and spirit. This system feeds, cleanses and heals the entire body.

One may experience multi-dimensional communion with spirit through acceleration of the lymphatic stream. The lymphatic white light system of spiritual healing facilitates bio-spiritual transformation. This technique is a holistic gateway to spirit. It is possible that the power of God can be manifested through the lymphatic system.

Lymph stream acceleration is defined as: The process of quickening the vital humors, energies of the body with the resultant therapeutic benefits of cleansing, nourishing, and rejuvenating on a systemic level.

Lymph stream acceleration is a dynamic, systemic, Massage of the whole person creating a unity of body humors or fluids and immune stimulation. Blood, sweat, tears, saliva, urine, mucus, cerebral spinal fluid, karyoplasm, cytoplasm, and digestive juices all develop from the embryonic sac of saline nutritive water into the lymphatic system and lymph fluids, which bring nutrition to the cellular level and health and immunity to the whole body.

The mother sea has spawned us creatures of crystallized minerals floating in liquid crystal water charged with bio-electric energy in perfect reflection of the cosmic sea. This is universal fact, why not use this knowledge consciously? The easy technique of lymph stream acceleration will put you into the flow of energy as Tai-Chi, yoga and meditation will make you more aware of the flow of energy. Lymph stream acceleration puts you directly in the flow by utilizing modalities to channel bio-electric energy combined with palmar massages of the connective tissue to accelerate and enhance the flow and function of the lymphatic system. This results in an increased cellular immunity (more white blood cells) and an increased humoral immunity (production of interferon and antibodies). Add to this the benefits of calming the nervous system and alleviating stress, and you have just a few of the many benefits of lymph stream acceleration. Lymph stream acceleration, a new approach to massage in the 21st century.

Lymphatic Massage is indicated for all people of all ages and is a very gentle, effective method of stress reduction and physical rejuvenation. The results gained with this technique cannot be replicated!

When discussing the dynamics of the lymphatic technique with students that have experienced the work, their descriptions were enlightening if not inspiring. Students gained a clear insight of the universal dynamic of the work. The fact that the technique is performed in wave-like spirals is key to the understanding of the power contained therein. The universe is constructed in circles or spirals. This creates what may be termed vortexian energy or cycloid space-curve motion, which is the motion of the planets, solar system, and galactic star systems. Indeed, this is the motion of the universe.

Understanding the true nature of the vortex may open the door to a new concept of the physical world and at the same time, open a gateway to the super physical world. The equivalence of matter and energy is not a new idea. The idea that a sub-atomic particle is a vortex of energy, as above so below, is a simple concept that has great power. The vortex demonstrates that apparently empty space is full of energy, and clarifies how energy relates to matter and how subtle energies such as the lymphatic spirals interact with the physical world. A resonance effect is created between these subtle energies and the energy in matter. Vortexes in air or water such as in the lymph stream, moving in the same form as the underlying energy in the universe may exchange energy with them. This principle may be demonstrated by two tuning forks in the same key creating a sympathetic vibration. This resonance effect may be a way of tapping into the cosmic energies of the universe itself. This could then facilitate spiritual evolution through the sympathetic effect created by the vortexian energy of the wave-like spirals used in Lymphatic Massage in toning and strengthening the immune system.

"Not as good as making love, but better than sex!" That's what one of my recent students said in reply to the question, "What does Lymphatic Massage feel like?" Clearly, he understood the exquisite pleasure to be had by merely relaxing, releasing and resolving. Relaxing clears physical stress, releasing clears psychological, emotional stress and resolving clears spiritual, cosmic, etheric stress as it were. But what about the part about making love?

"Is love not a part of healing?" I asked. "Oh, yes of course," he replied, "but you asked what it felt like, and it feels better than sex, but not as good as making love!" Yet when the technique is done correctly, not only does the client receiving the treatment feel the exquisite pleasure of the gentle, loving touch, but everyone in the room is affected by the powerful, energetic aspect of this spiritual art. Lymphatic Massage could put you in touch with all that there is in existence, or at least help you gain a better insight as you progress on your path to enlightenment.

The ancient Chinese stated that the spirit is carried in the Chi and the Chi is carried in the lymph stream. The joy of Lymphatic Massage is that since the lymph runs under the skin, when we touch the skin to accelerate the lymph flow, we do indeed lay hands on spirit!

What a wonderful art for couples to learn. In fact everyone can benefit from learning a new age way of touching that heals! Come share God's love and light in healing the living waters of the planet and ourselves with Lymphatic Massage.

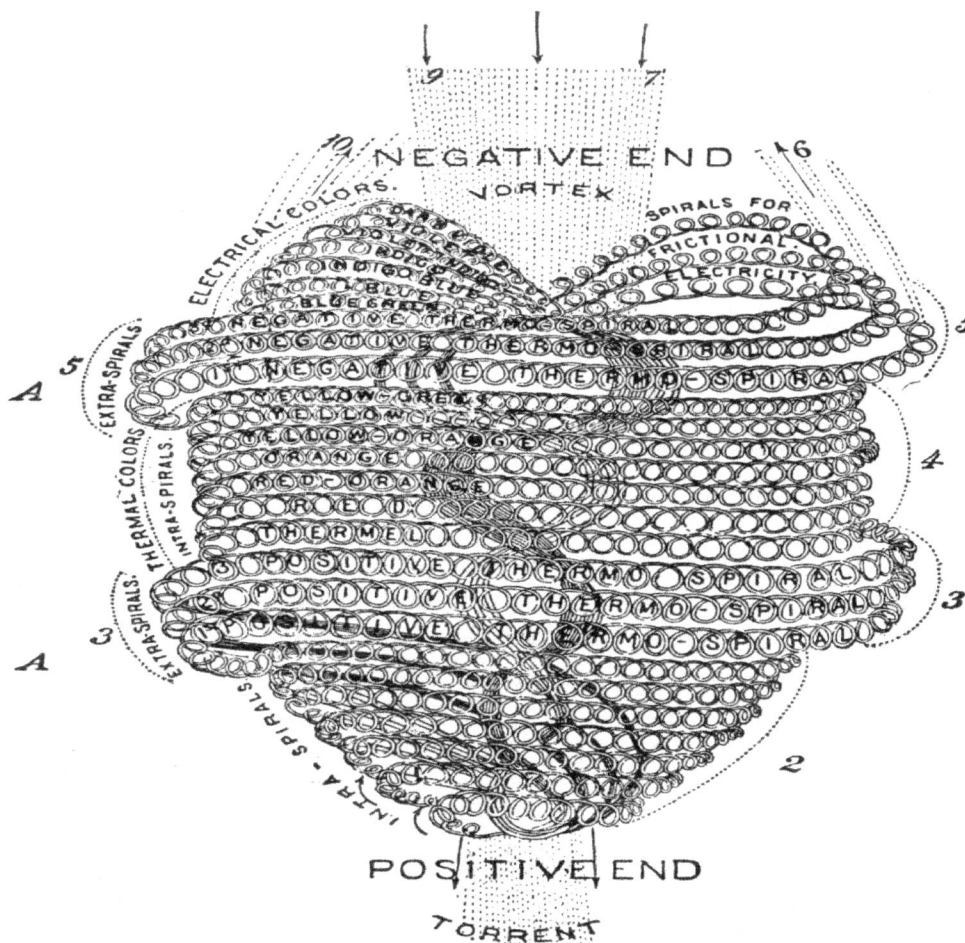

From Babbitt's *Principles of Light and Color.*

THE LYMPHATIC SYSTEM:
PHYSICAL HEALTH AND SPIRITUAL COMMUNION

Since our homeostatic and defense mechanisms work below our levels of perception, most often we are unaware of the struggle that is constantly going on in our body. All of the foreign materials that we inhale, ingest or absorb by contact are a threat to us and must be neutralized. Beyond that, we must maintain a constant internal milieu for the cell population. Therefore, any drastic change in our environmental or chemical interface (diet) must be met with prompt and vigorous action on the part of our homeostatic mechanisms. Understanding this, one might conclude that most of our illnesses are homeostatic dysfunctions, that is our inability to cope with stressors.

Most people will vary their stress threshold. On our better times, when we eat and rest well, have low levels of stress, to raise the level of coping beyond normal is a significant task and one that can only be done at a fundamental, even perhaps a spiritual level. It is a current wide spread fallacy that good nutrition and exercise alone put one in an optimal state of health. Not that these efforts are not important, they are, but we do have an upper limit dictated by our original genetic liability and irreversible degeneration. There are some techniques that can alter this picture. The massage of the lymphatic system is an ancient process that has a significant impact on our level of stress, and therefore the development of our spirituality.

The lymphatic system is one of the basic systems that effects everything in the body. It effects the defense and homeostatic systems. In the defense system, it is part of the immune system, and in homeostasis, it helps maintain the correct environment for all the cells to thrive. See Figure (1) for the lymphatic system's effect on the nutritional gradient flow system necessary for cell health.

One of the functions of the lymphatic system is to balance the pressure between the fluid compartments of the cells (extracellular, intracellular, etc.). When the lymphatic system backs up, because of blockage, pressure builds up in the lymph capillary, and then in the cell bed. This causes a loss of a necessary pressure gradient which allows substances to move from the blood compartment to the cell bed, therefore cells fail to get their necessary nutrients and other molecules. Beyond that, the cell bed becomes toxic due to waste disposal failure. Cells, under these conditions, frequently lose metabolic efficiency, and therefore fail to do their assigned jobs well. If enough cells are in this state, the patient loses energy and feels poorly. The spaces between the cells are known as the interstitial spaces. These spaces are filled with water and other constituents such as colloids, fibers and other molecules that wander through these spaces such as vitamins, minerals, nutrients and hormones. The balance between liquids and solids determines the mobility of the nutrients among the cells. During fluid shifts such as edema and dehydration, the passage of those constituents may be impaired. (See Figure 2)

Dr. William N. Brown Ph.D., N.D., D.Sc.

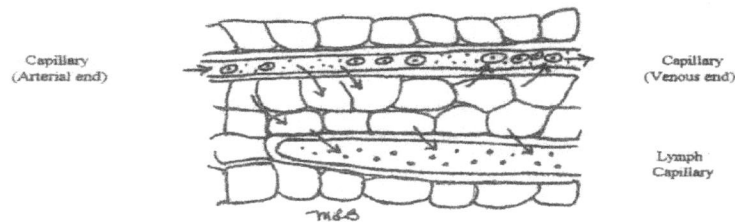

Capillary
(Arterial end)

Capillary
(Venous end)

Lymph
Capillary

Fluid Exchange - It appears that such large molecules as proteins (black dots) and lipids (open circles) leave the blood capillaries along with the fluid and salts. Some of the fluid and salts are reabsorbed; the excess, alone with large molecules that cannot re-enter the blood capillaries, is returned via the lymphatic system.

Fig. 1

Substances leave capillaries because of a net effective hydrostatic pressure; other substances enter the capillaries because of a net effective osmotic pressure.

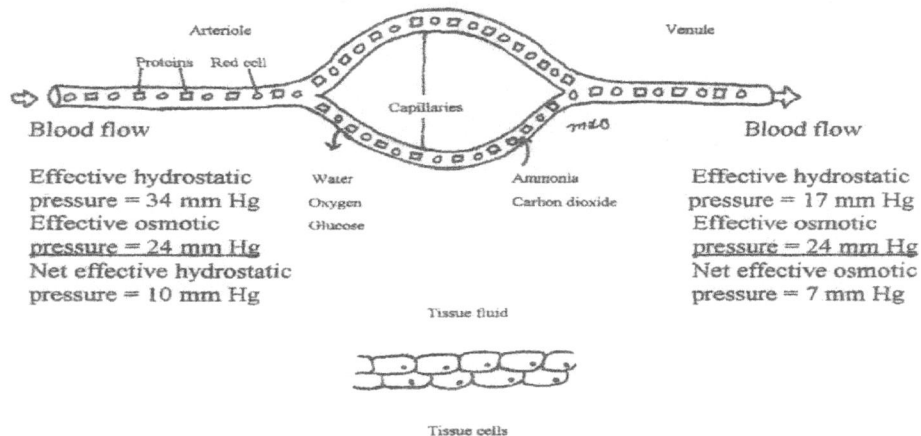

Arteriole

Venule

Proteins   Red cell

Capillaries

Blood flow

Blood flow

Effective hydrostatic
pressure = 34 mm Hg
Effective osmotic
pressure = 24 mm Hg
Net effective hydrostatic
pressure = 10 mm Hg

Water   Ammonia
Oxygen   Carbon dioxide
Glucose

Effective hydrostatic
pressure = 17 mm Hg
Effective osmotic
pressure = 24 mm Hg
Net effective osmotic
pressure = 7 mm Hg

Tissue fluid

Tissue cells

Fig. 2

People in general understand the need and actions of the blood system in the body. However, the lymph system, which is the second system of circulation, is poorly understood by both doctors and laymen alike. Every health professional learns about the presence of the system in school, but it is usually a brief mention and even then the focus is on pathology, such as cancer or severe lymphadenopathies like elephantiasis.

To understand why and how the lymph system develops problems, a brief description is in order. Everywhere from head to toe, that there is a blood capillary, there is a lymph capillary. Unfortunately, for the most part, the system drains into the venous blood (its final destination) only at the right and left subclavian veins. This means that even if some waste starts its journey in the big toe, it must travel through the whole body before it can escape into the subclavian. Even though it may be classified as the third system of circulation, its pattern is considerably different from the first two (arterial and venous). The lymph system's pattern is more like that of a railroad system, that is to say, there are tracts (lymph channels) going toward central yards (lymph nodes) and from there, to more central ducts (such as the thoracic) and then out. To go on to the why, if the system contains more than it can easily handle, various molecules and substances may coalesce at a narrowing point, such as an entry into a node. They may then form an obstruction or block to continued flow. Since the system is rather flexible, any following substances will seek collateral circulation. (See Figure 3)

LYMPHATIC NODE

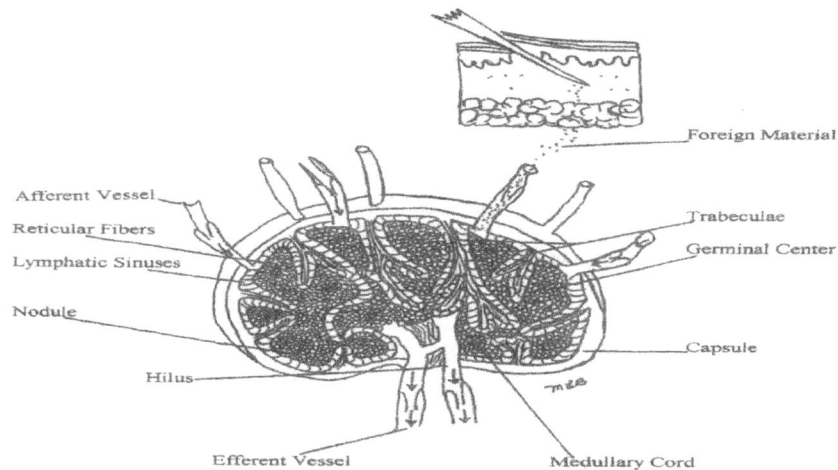

Fig. 3

Over the years, the Lymphatic Massage techniques have been developed to promote lymph flow. To understand why traditional massage fails to help in many cases, I would like to use the following analogy. Imagine if you fill a funnel with sand, or for the purpose of this illustration, glass beads, and leave the particles loose, the material will flow. If you try to shove the particles through, they will jam up. The more pressure you apply, the worse the problem becomes. The effect of the Lymphatic Massage will be to charge the particles so that they repel each other, thereby separating and re-establishing the flow. Then with the gentle urging of the Lymphatic Massage one may accelerate the flow of the lymph stream. This is a very simple explanation of what is a much more complex biochemically therapeutic event, and a spiritual alignment energetically.

Figure 4 represents a view of some of the general flow patterns of the lymphatic system. I should mention that Lymphatic Massage will be discussed in regard to the immune system,

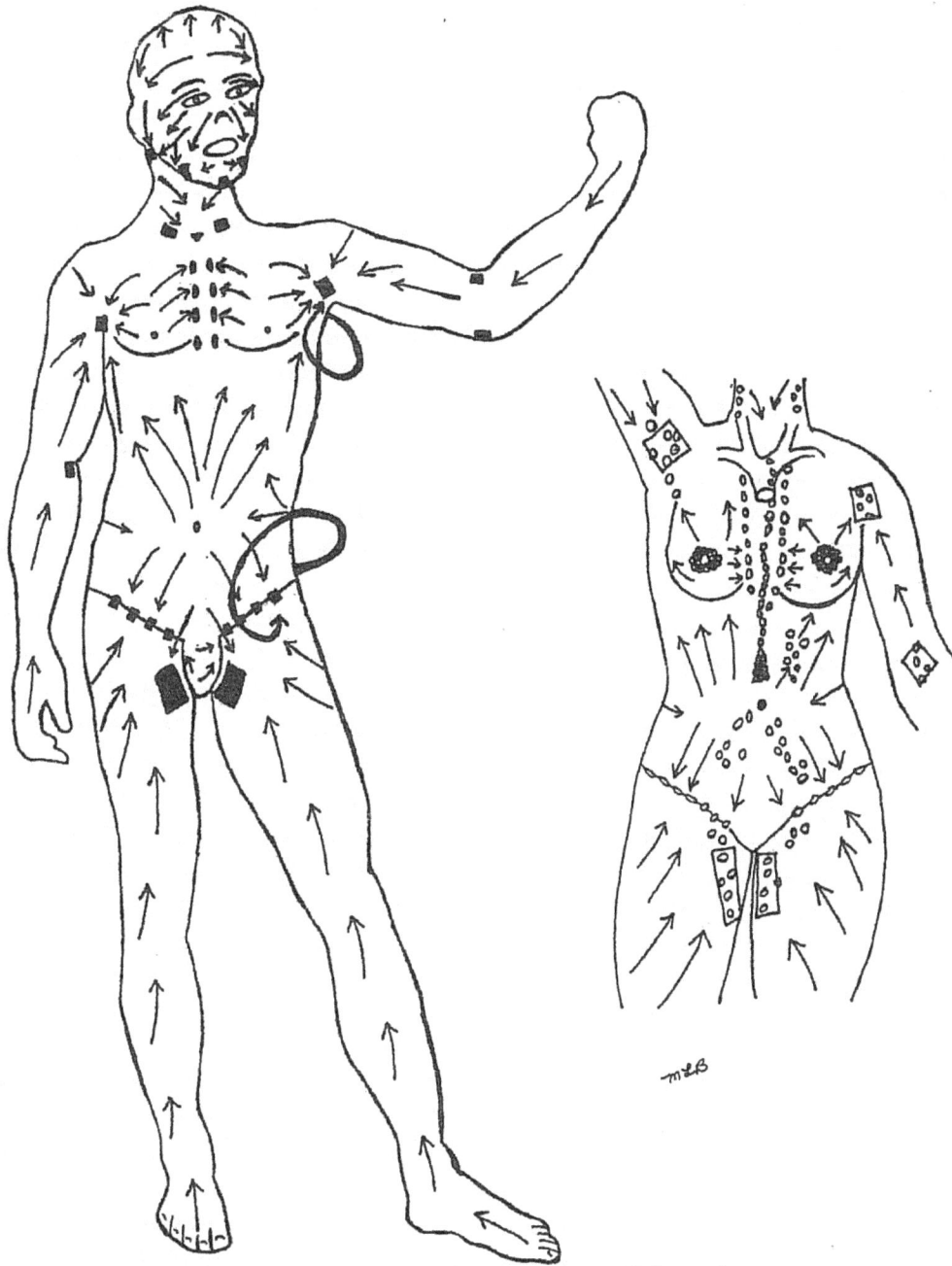

Fig. 4

which is an integral part of the lymphatics. As you can see, the flow, in general is upward, with the exception of the head and areas near major lymph node centers. The head and neck are areas where people often first notice lymphatic problems. Especially with children, swollen nodes under the jaw and near the ears are common occurrences. Other major node groups are shown in the axilla (arm pit) and the lower abdomen (groin). Some small nodes reside in the extremities as shown here in the arm. There are many more deep nodes than there are superficial ones, and the intestinal tract has a significant number.

Since women are more responsive to internal hormonal flows, lymphatic problems are more apparent. Women suffer problems at the rate of 8 to 10 times that of men. One of the reasons is that excessive female hormones tend to aggravate any predisposition one might have. This may occur with some oral contraceptives, especially if poorly prescribed. A hormone depressing drug (Danazole) tends to help in some cases, but it is temporary. It may also have significant adverse side effects. Then too, females seen to have thirst perversions at a rate much higher than men which causes them to suffer from borderline dehydration. Females that present with these conditions seldom drink much water and often speak of their dislike for the taste of it. Very often, the first presenting symptom will be tenderness around the breast especially just before her period. The breast is particularly vulnerable since it is made of passive tissue (adipose and glandular) and therefore must be drained by osmotic force, whereas the muscle movement forces fluid flow in most other tissue. (See Figure 5).

A series of one way valves, much like those found in the venous system prevent the return of the lymphatic fluid toward gravity. That is why exercise is so useful. In sedentary people, the lymph tens to stagnate in about twenty minutes. To some degree after that, the cells are exposed to their own toxic waste. The acceleration of breathing rapidly pushes on the thoracic duct that lies on the inner aspect of the spine, increasing flow and almost acting as a pump for the rest of the system. The exception to this is when the lymph system is blocked in certain areas, exercise will increase metabolic waste which then will tend to accumulate distal to (beyond) the blocked area where it will be difficult to remove. Accumulations of this type are what have been referred to as "CELLULITE". Initially, these infiltrates are strictly fluid waste, but after a long period, if the situation is not corrected, fibrosis sets in. At that time, the condition is much harder and time consuming to treat. Diet can and often does contribute to the problem. Caffeine is a potent enemy of the lymphatic system. This is why many physicians recommend removing all caffeine from the diet of women with fibrocystic breast disease. Many studies have shown this correlation. Using diet modulation and Lymphatic Massage, it has been demonstrated in many cases that the condition resolves itself without any other invasive intervention.

Beyond this, high fat, high protein diets tend to cause problems in the lymph system. The incomplete digestion of proteins result in absorption of peptides and other debris in the process of metabolism. Fats from the intestinal tract are absorbed into the blood through the lacteals which are part of the lymph system. If the system is at all compromised, heavy fat intake makes it all the more sluggish. However, through the technique of Lymphatic Massage, the molecular structure of fat in the lymph stream is changed from gelatinous to liquid, and the sluggish lymph stream is accelerated.

THE LYMPHATIC SYSTEM

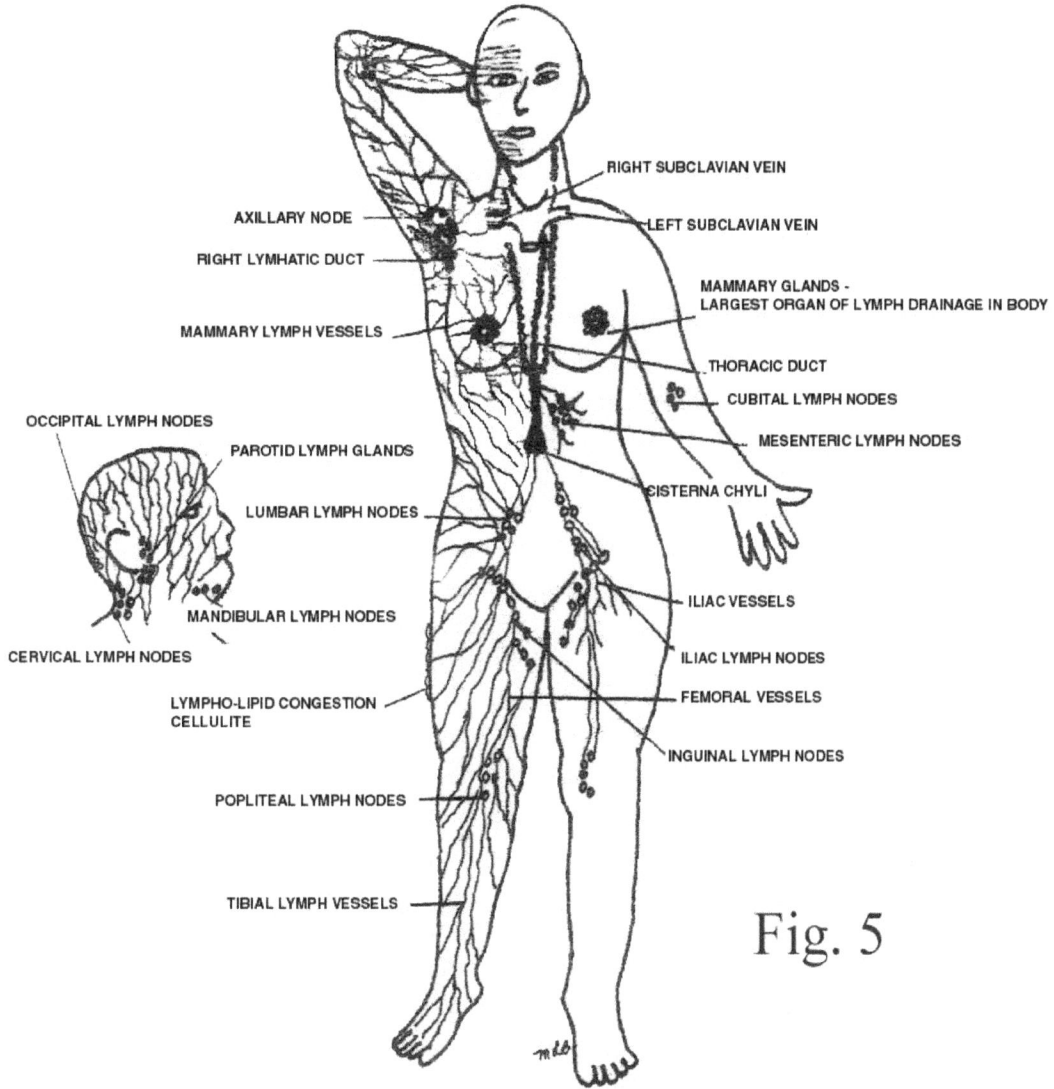

RIGHT SUBCLAVIAN VEIN

AXILLARY NODE

LEFT SUBCLAVIAN VEIN

RIGHT LYMHATIC DUCT

MAMMARY GLANDS - LARGEST ORGAN OF LYMPH DRAINAGE IN BODY

MAMMARY LYMPH VESSELS

THORACIC DUCT

CUBITAL LYMPH NODES

OCCIPITAL LYMPH NODES

MESENTERIC LYMPH NODES

PAROTID LYMPH GLANDS

CISTERNA CHYLI

LUMBAR LYMPH NODES

ILIAC VESSELS

MANDIBULAR LYMPH NODES

ILIAC LYMPH NODES

CERVICAL LYMPH NODES

FEMORAL VESSELS

LYMPHO-LIPID CONGESTION CELLULITE

INGUINAL LYMPH NODES

POPLITEAL LYMPH NODES

TIBIAL LYMPH VESSELS

Fig. 5

Vessels in shaded area drain into right lymphatic duct.
All other vessels drain into thoracic duct.

Appetite perversions occur due to the breakdown in the pressure gradient which impedes the flow of nutrients to the cells, causing such things as sweet cravings. The abdomen is literally filled with lymph networks which help keep the intestinal tissue in a healthy state. Colitis is an inflammation of the large bowel or colon. In treating this condition, it has been found that the bowel will not heal as long as the lymphatic channels coming from it are blocked. As soon as they are cleared, the case is quickly resolved.

The diet that seems to have proven best over time is the high complex carbohydrate, low fat, low protein diet. This seems to have a cleansing effect, decreases the transit time (food going through the tract faster) and keeps the bowel bacteria healthier. This latter consideration is proving to be perhaps the major reason this type of diet contributes to preventing colon cancer, since dying bacteria produce a carcinogenic residue that may cause colon cancer.

Observation of lymphatic problems is a quick and easy process. Two things are involved. Knowing where to locate indicator points, and second, the feel or texture of the tissue under consideration. Figure 6 is a front (anterior) view and a back (posterior) view with noted areas where lymph problems occur. Further on in the text, more details will be given as to specific location and significance of what is found on palpation of the point.

To palpate, flat fingers are used to put light circular pressure at a 45 degree angle over the desired area to determine the texture of the tissue (IE. soft and puffy, hard and ropy, dry and sandy etc.). Usually you will be able to notice the difference and the treatment can progress. In some areas, you will be dependent on the person's response, in other places you will be able to tell by the feel of the tissue. It will take awhile to determine the difference between normal and abnormal tissue. Some people are firmer while others are softer in general. In muscle you will find that tissue that is infiltrated with waste will be ropy or stiffened. Such tissue cannot drain properly and will, as a result feel uncomfortable when palpated. Often, people with lymphatic problems have a characteristic turgid or swollen feel to their tissue. They tend to carry extra fluids (and thereby weight) which can be noticed before the Lymphatic Massage is begun.

Hormonal and metabolic problems or the tendency to these problems need not be genetic. They can be acquired with age. General abuse and environmental insults, bad diet, stress and other factors play a role in such acquisitions. Certain disease, infections, and inflammatory responses will cause acute as well as chronic problems. In addition to this, trauma from accidents, burns as well as surgical interventions may cause temporary or permanent injury to the tissue for obvious reasons. Other miscellaneous cause, such as dehydration, alcohol and drug abuse, tight or restrictive clothing like wired bras, etc. that interfere with easy flow of the body's superficial fluid pathways, certain prescribed medications such as oral contraceptives, and dietary indiscretions as previously mentioned, may all play a role in lymphatic problems.

Due to the mind body connection, problems which manifest in the body are related to energetic imbalances. The release or clearing of the problems in one area affects the other and vice versa. The lymphatic system can be viewed energetically as a bridge that spans the third and fourth dimension. When the lymph stream is properly accelerated through the Lymphatic Massage, it exhibits all the phenomena of time space relationships, which is fourth dimensional, and hence, the connection with spirit.

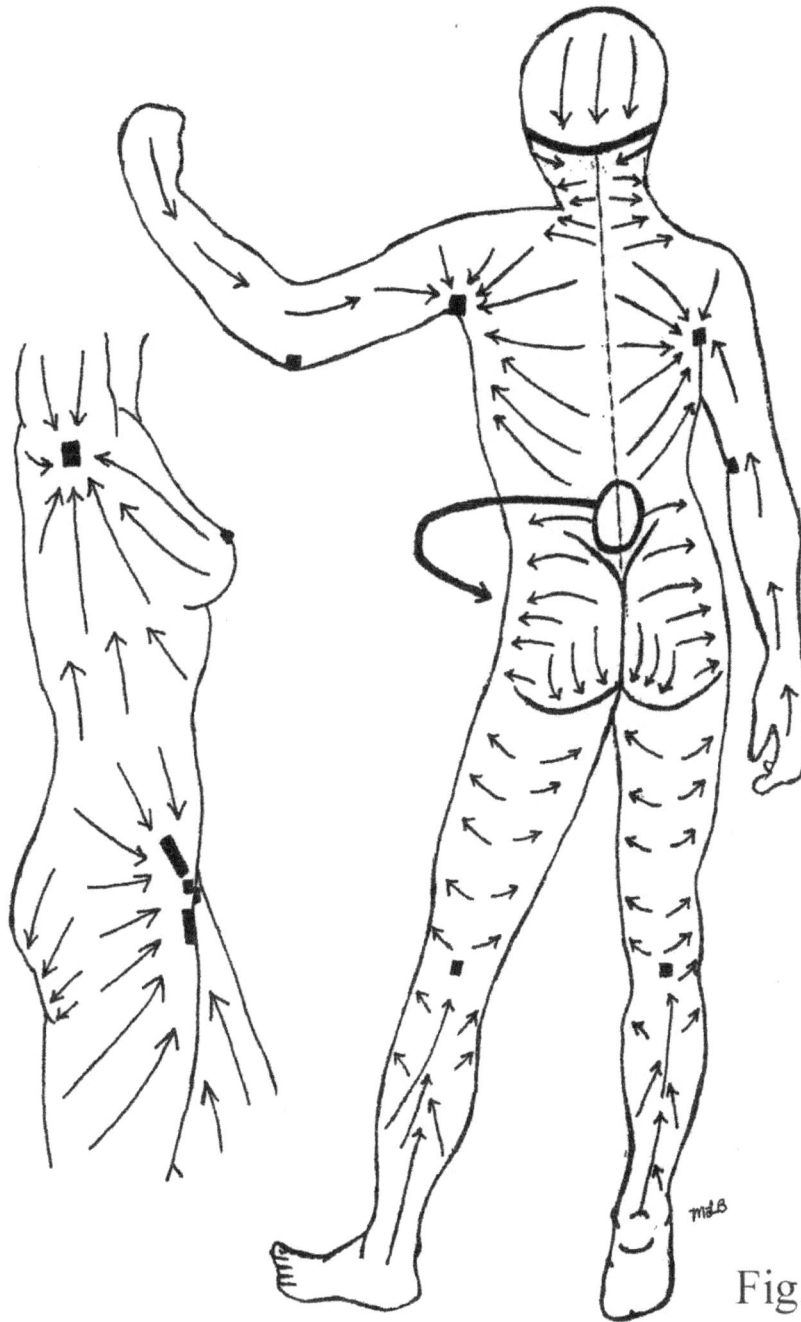

Fig. 6

Since the endocrine system secretes its hormones directly into lymph and controls hormonal balance physically, energetically the endocrine system relates to the chakras, and therefore to spiritual balance. The acceleration of the life stream (lymph stream) through the Lymphatic Massage makes clear the relationship between physical, emotional, and spiritual balance. It has been said that God's love is expressed through creation as touch. If this is true, then the power of God's love can be felt in the immune system. (See Figure 7)

Since our lymphatic system is our immune system, the cleansing and toning of our lymphatic system provides the benefit of a responsive immune system. Due to the fact that the energetic must exist before the physical, or as it was once stated, "as above, so below". When balance is achieved on a physical level, balance is also achieved energetically. It is the energetic aspect of the Lymphatic Massage that allows for the spiritual application of the work.

It is the emotional and psychological aspect of the life stream acceleration that supports the spiritual evolution of Humanity. Through the Lymphatic Massage we provide a nurturing environment for the accelerated spiritual development of mankind. From cell to spirit, the lymphatic system is the hidden door to the kingdom of God within.

This white light technique promotes the union of self with the living, loving, healing God within the body temple. It has been theorized that the power of God is contained within the lymphatic system, because this is the system of the body which heals, nourishes, and cleanses on the cellular level. Lymphatic Massage is therefore a spiritual art of healing which utilizes the principles of Christ consciousness.

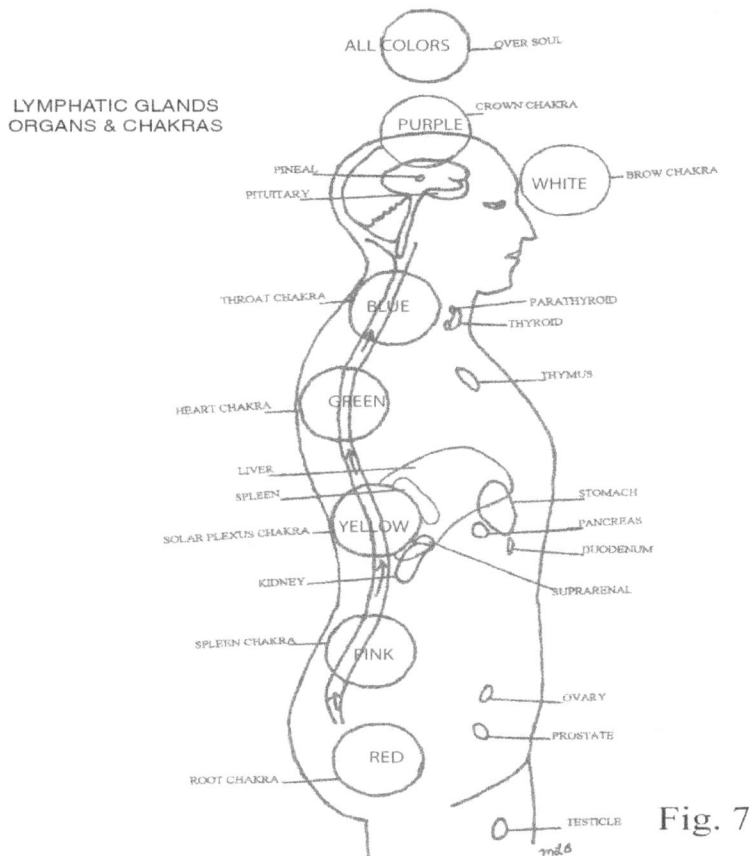

LYMPHATIC GLANDS
ORGANS & CHAKRAS

ALL COLORS — OVER SOUL

CROWN CHAKRA

PURPLE

PINEAL

PITUITARY

WHITE — BROW CHAKRA

THROAT CHAKRA — BLUE — PARATHYROID / THYROID

THYMUS

HEART CHAKRA — GREEN

LIVER

SPLEEN — STOMACH

SOLAR PLEXUS CHAKRA — YELLOW — PANCREAS / DUODENUM

KIDNEY — SUPRARENAL

SPLEEN CHAKRA — PINK

OVARY

PROSTATE

RED

ROOT CHAKRA

TESTICLE

Fig. 7

This lymphatic art is a very ancient and unique white light method of spiritual healing. It is energetic bodywork which allows you to come into communion with your higher self through lymphatic purification.

Cleanliness is next to Godliness, and through the white light, heart chakra energy balancing system of Lymphatic Massage, peace and wholeness are achieved in mind, body and spirit. The Lymphatic Massage is the holistic gateway to the realm of the spirit, which can help you open yourself to the free flow of spirit within and truly enter the kingdom of God. It allows you to experience multidimensional communion with spirit. (See figure 8) This magical method of healing is bio-spiritual transformation in preparation for ascension and the nurturing embrace of spirit, here and now!

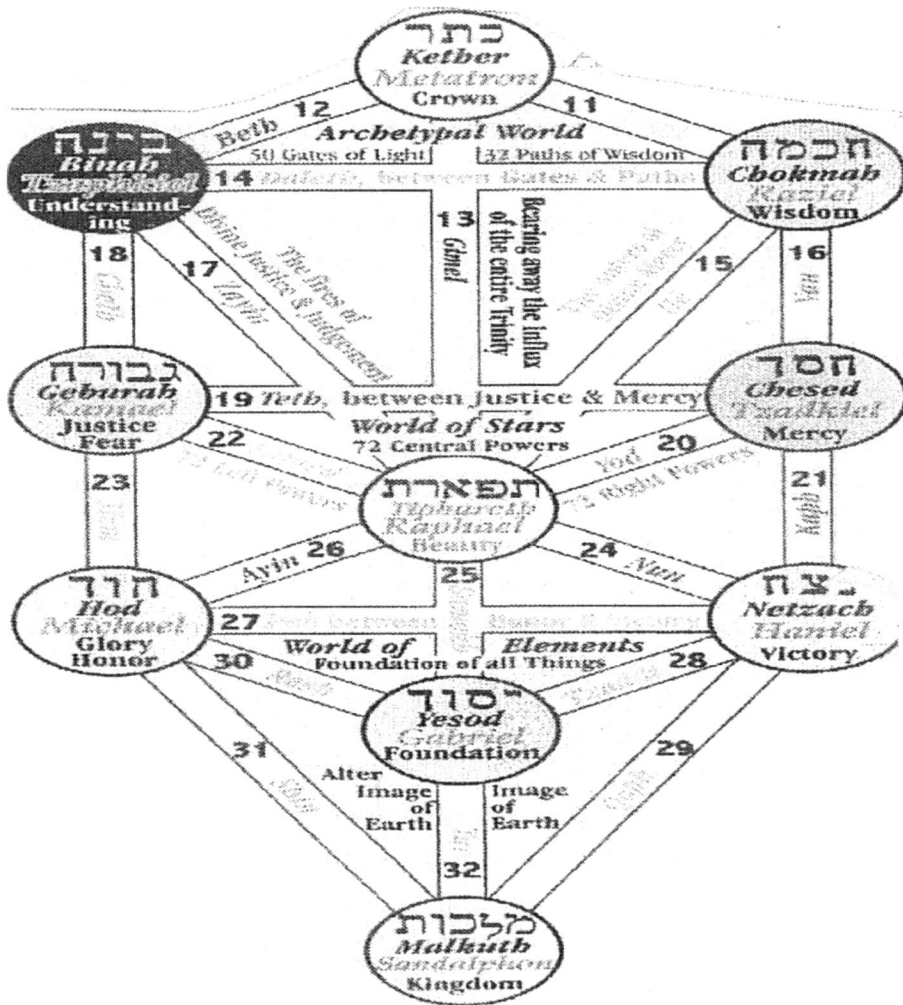

Fig. 8

"The lymphatic principles, he who knows these understandingly, possesses the magic key before whose touch, all doors of the body temple fly open."

Adapted from
The Kybalion

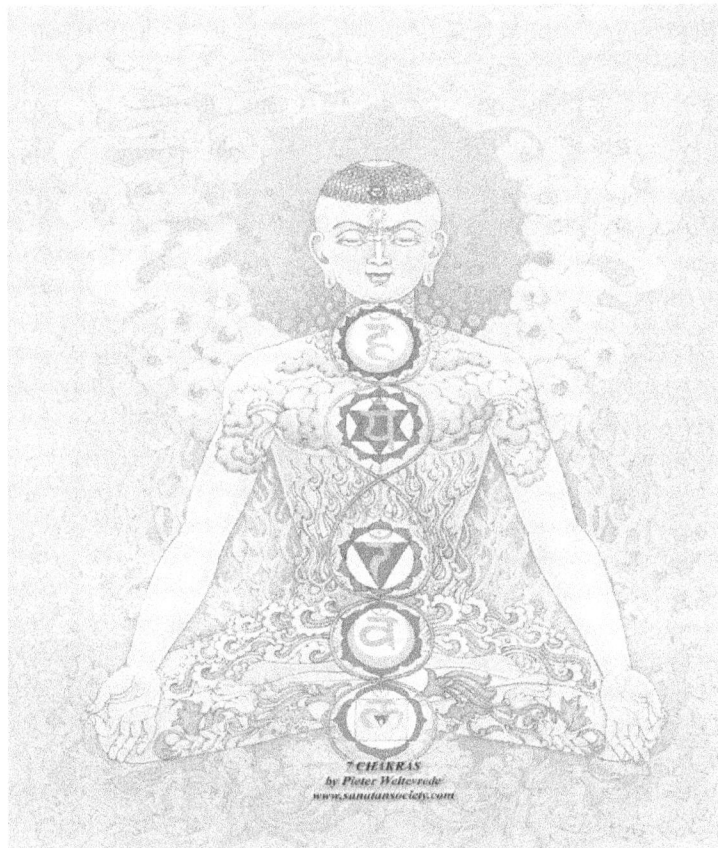

7 CHAKRAS
by Pieter Weltevrede
www.sanatansociety.com

PART TWO

THE GROUNDING TECHNIQUE

The *grounding technique*, as taught by Dr. Brown, is a dynamic creative visualization designed to protect, direct, and control the energy flow of the practitioner to the patient.

First, you visualize white light coming directly from the heart of God, down through your crown, past your throat and into your heart chakra. Then see the white light as it moves into your shoulders, arms and hands and over the person on the table; filing the entire room with white light. Next, you visualize your connection with the very center of the earth, and visualize the energy of the earth spiraling around you as the white light flows down and through you. Set your intention through prayer as follows:

> *"Dear Father-Mother God, I thank you for allowing me to be your*
> *instrument of healing, to heal this person for their highest good."*

Finally, you incorporate the pranic yoga breath with the kabalistic technique of soohan or 'bringing down the light'. This is the grounding technique instituted before you ever touch the patient.

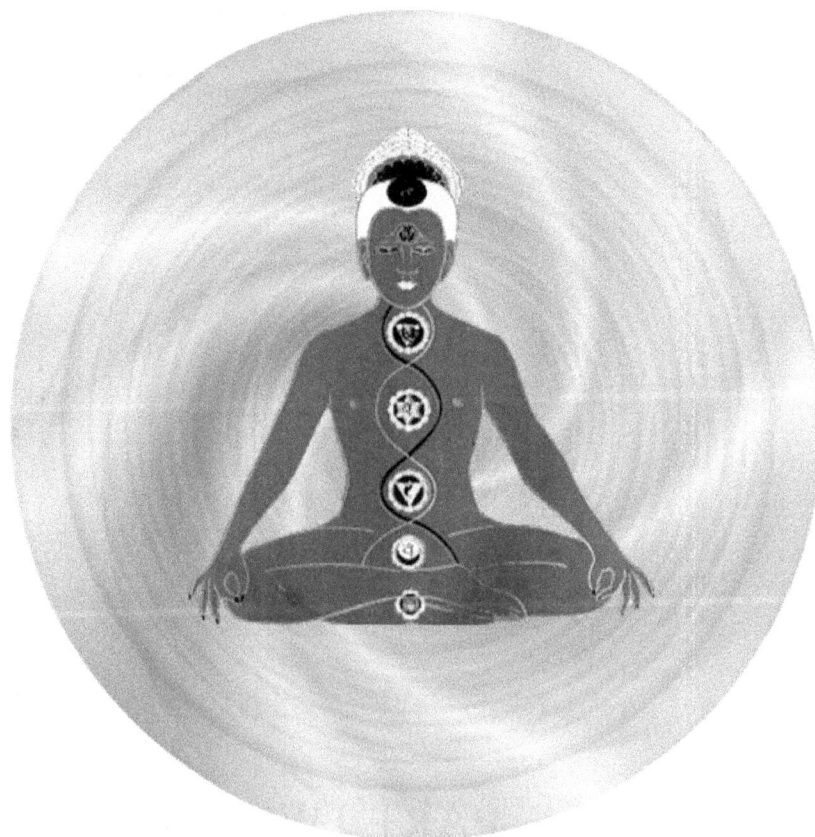

VISUALIZATION OF THE GROUNDING TECHNIQUE

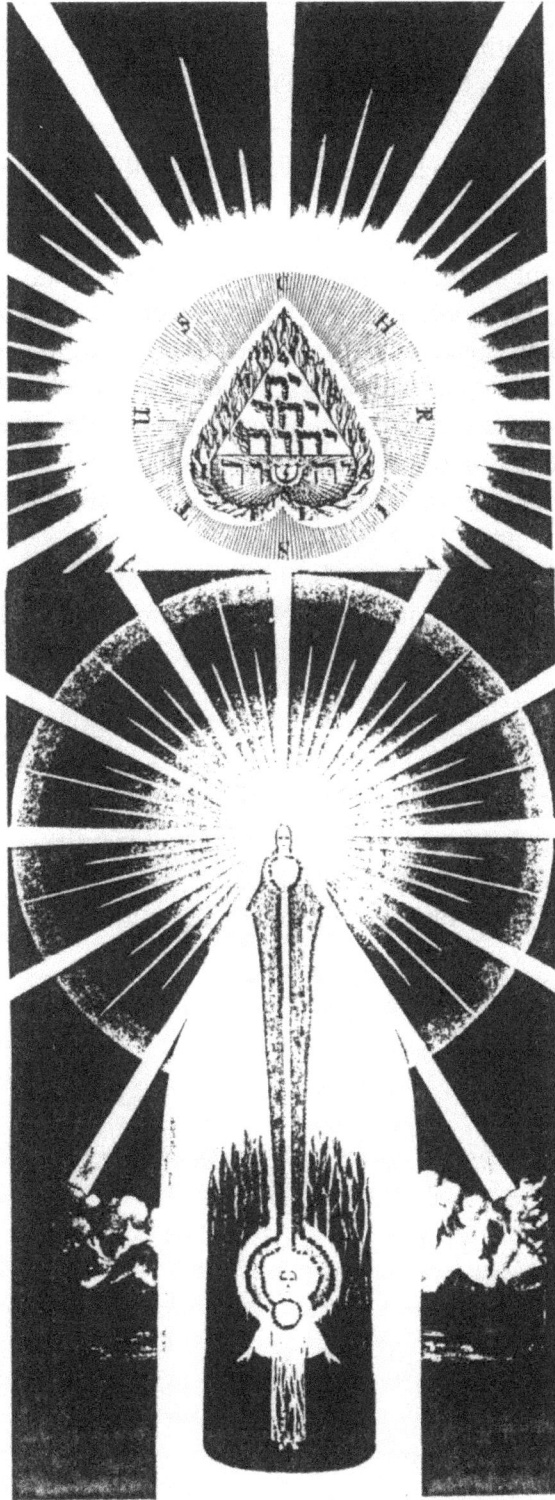

THE LYMPHATIC MASSAGE TECHNIQUE

A Neo-Vodderian Method of Manual Lymph Drainage

This method is a synthesis of bio-energetic hand manipulations of the lymphatic system, after the technique of William N. Brown, Ph.D.

Before touching the client, <u>always</u> apply proper grounding techniques to establish energy flow.

The first movement is an effleurage over the pectoralis, starting at midstream and moving to the acromion process. Next, circles at the sternal notch. Thumb circles around the base of the neck, starting at the medial aspect o the clavicle to the 7th cervical vertebrae and returning to the starting point. Work the clavicular hollow from medial to lateral, ending again at the acromion process. Pivot the hands on the thumbs bringing the four flat fingers to the occiput, work from the base of the skull in a circular motion, down the neck. Use the webbing of the hand to do a superficial friction over the superior aspect of the trapezius, from medial to lateral and from later to medial. Then pull the traps.

Instruct the client to arch spine, position hands under spine, then client relaxes. To work spine, use fingers to circle toward spine, then lifts three times upward, working from waist up. Roll the traps.

Work the neck from the angle of the jaw to the base of the neck.. Circles at the sternal notch, circles under the medial aspect of the lower mandible with one finger, then all fingers under mandible, to the angle of jaw* to temples* (*facial circuit). Work the top of the chin from medial to lateral and do facial circuit. Feel for energy at corner of the eyes. Do the top lip with circles going toward midline of lip, then move laterally with circles going toward little fingers and do facial circuit.

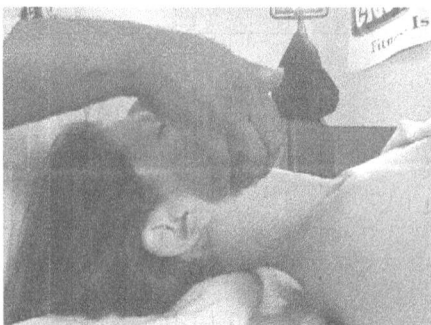
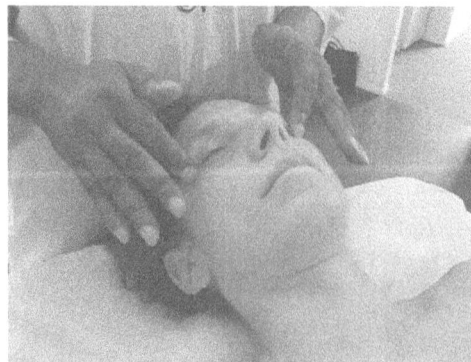

Circle under eyes from lateral to medial, stroke *over* the gabella. Work the nose, then do facial circuit. Repeat circles under eyes and gabella strokes.

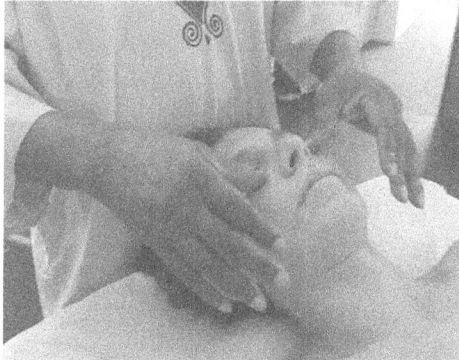

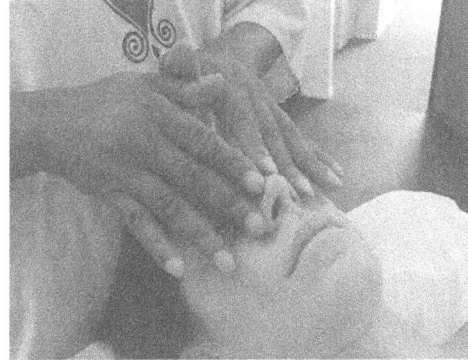

Wrinkle the right eyebrow, repeat circles under eyes and gabella strokes. Wrinkle the left eyebrow, repeat circles under eyes and gabella strokes. Wrinkle both eyebrows simultaneously, repeat circles under eyes and gabella strokes.

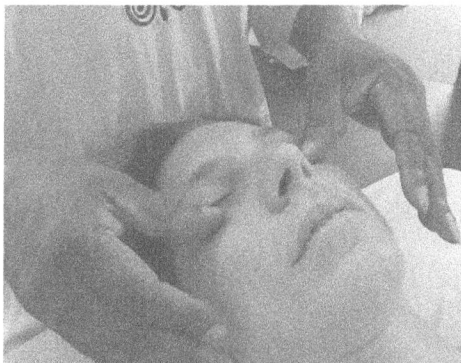

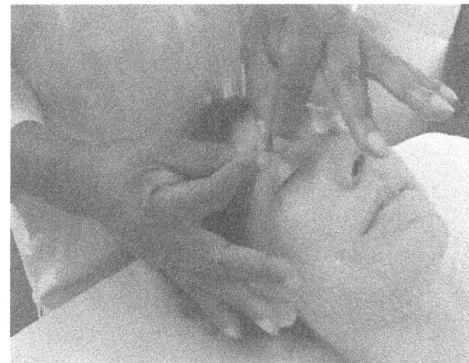

Do stationary circles on lacrimeal duct. Do stationary circles over third eye. Do stationary circles with four flat fingers over forehead. Thumb slides over forehead.

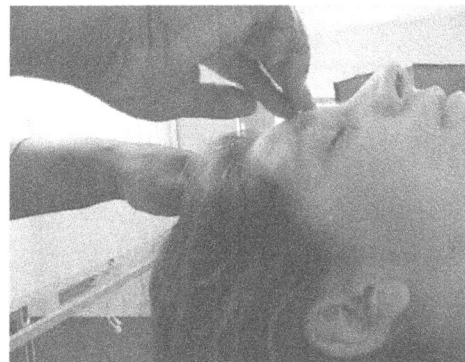

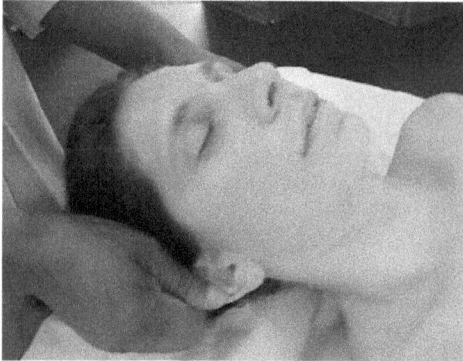

Work the scalp. Work ears - squeeze from bottom to top, insert finger into ear openings and do rotations. Squeeze the tragus, the do ear pulls and stationary circles under the ears.

Move to the right side of the table, thumb slides across left side of face. Circles under left side of mandible from medial to lateral, ending at ear. Move to left side of table and repeat process on right side of face. Move to head of table and circles down neck toward clavicle.

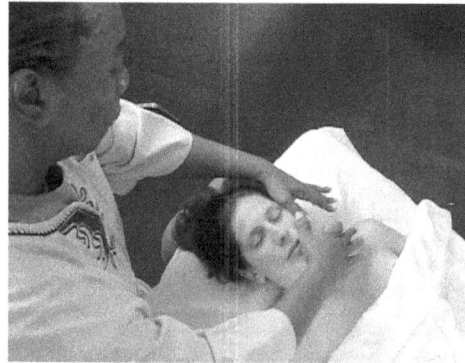

Do effleurage over chest, chin, cheeks, and forehead.

Move to left side, do circles in axilla with four flat fingers. Shake arm from distal to proximal and lay arm down.

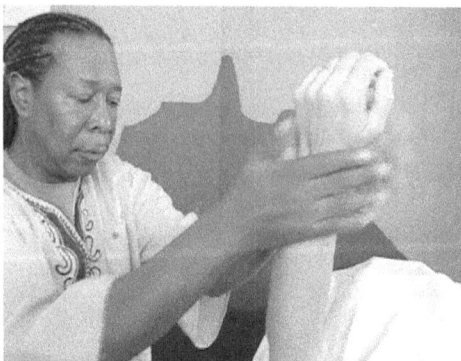

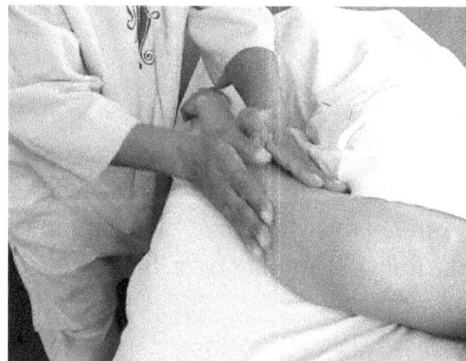

Push-pull proximal to distal and distal to proximal, Choo-choo proximal to distal and distal to proximal. Choo-choo from shoulder to elbow, circles on elbow, choo-choo to wrist.

Spread hand, squeeze webbing between fingers and thumb, circles between metacarpals to wrist, milk the fingers. Squeeze fingers and thumb to palm, circles on palm, squeeze palm to wrist, rotate wrist. Scoob from shoulder to elbow, scoob from elbow to wrist, scoob from wrist to elbow, then one-handed scoob from elbow to shoulder. Lift arm and squeeze down, lay arm down and effleurage distal to proximal.

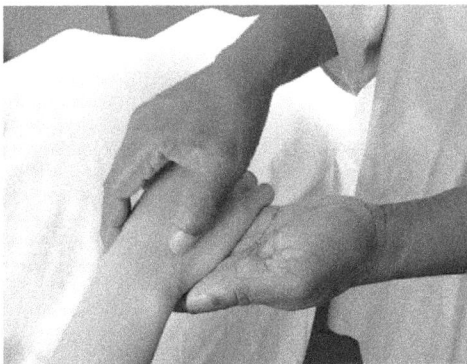

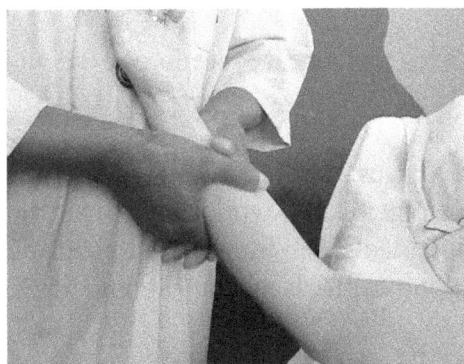

Pump left breast, circles on breast with four flat fingers, rotate breast. Circle diagonally across body to right hip. Circles around the abdomen.

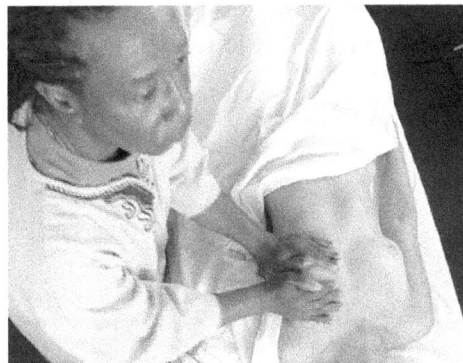

Move to right leg. Work right inner thigh and inquinal area with stationary circles. Circles along inquinal fold. Rock leg at pelvis and knee, then knee and instep, then back to pelvis and knee. Shake leg proximal to distal, then distal to proximal.

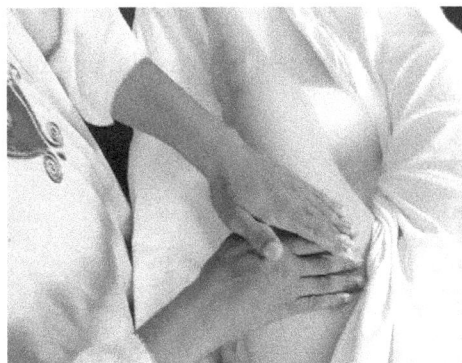

Push-pull proximal to distal, then distal to proximal. Choo-choo proximal to distal, and distal to proximal. Scoob from thigh to knee. Thumb circles across ankle, lateral to medial then medial to lateral. Rotate foot. Pump ankles. Scoob up leg to pelvis, then diagonally across the body to left axilla.

Move to right arm and repeat procedures used on left arm.

Move to head of table, both hands circles down both sides of sternum, (circle in toward sternum), then finger circles in intercostals from inferior to superior, ending at axilla.

Move to right breast and repeat procedures used on left breast.

Move to left leg and repeat procedures used on right leg.

Raise knees. Shake left calf, pat calf. Inverted scoob from ankle to knee, work knee. Shake left thigh, pat thigh. Inverted scoob from ankle to gluteals. Work inguinal and gluteal folds meeting at hip. Move to right leg and repeat process.

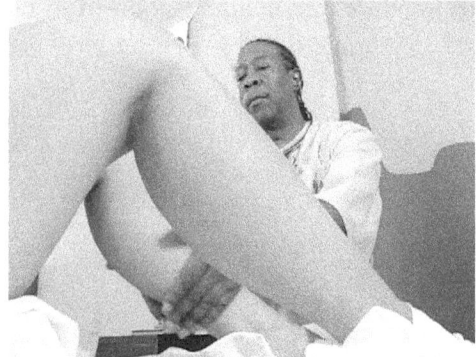

Firm circles over abdominal area with knees bent. Lower legs. Scoob left side of body (medial to lateral) from ankle to axilla.

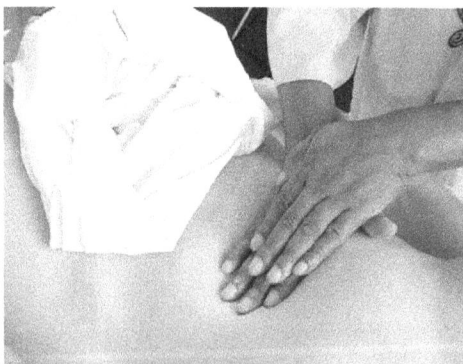

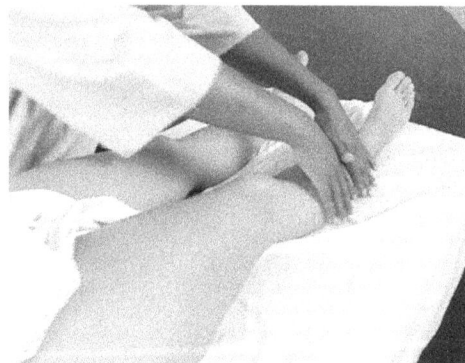

Scallop left side from ankle to axilla, ending with circles at axial. Repeat procedure in right side. Effleurage.

Instruct client to turn away from therapist, onto abdomen with arms on table at sides. Work the scalp. Cranial squeezes. Vibrate at occiput. Scoob back of neck. Finger circles on sides of cervical vertebrae, pop neck.

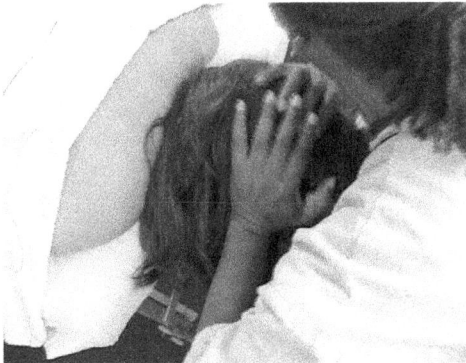

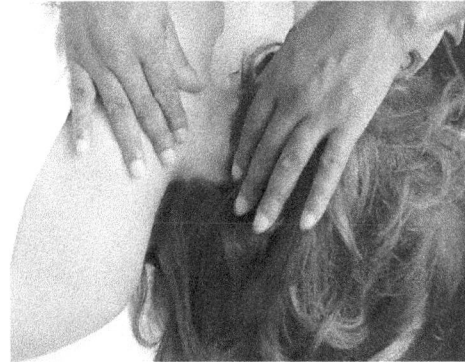

Finger circles on scalp. Flat finger circles on sides of neck. Thumb circles on traps. Trap twists with pumps on left shoulder, repeat on right shoulder. Circles down spine (in toward spine) to waist and finger circles in intercostals to axilla. Monkey climbing left side of back, waist to shoulder, then right side, then over spine. Inchworm up back from waist to shoulders.

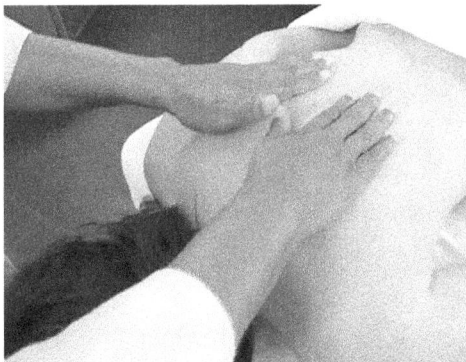

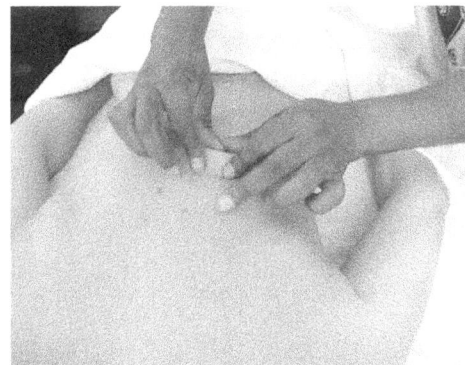

Pump left gluteal, kneading then fulling. Circles on gluteal, work gluteal fold. Shake left leg, proximal to distal, distal to proximal. Push-pull proximal to distal, distal to proximal. Choo-choo proximal to distal, distal to proximal. Scoob from gluteal to popliteal space, circles on popliteal space. Scoob to ankle. Reflexology on foot. Pump ankles. Scoob from ankle to axilla. Move to right side a repeat procedures used on left gluteal and leg.

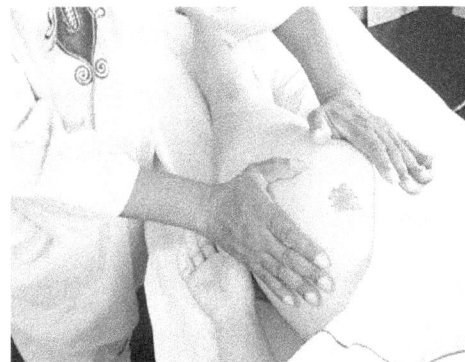

Scoob left side of body (medial to lateral) from ankle to axilla. Scallop left side from ankle to axilla. Kidney pumps. Scoob from waist to axilla, scallop from ankle to axilla. Repeat above procedures on right side of body.

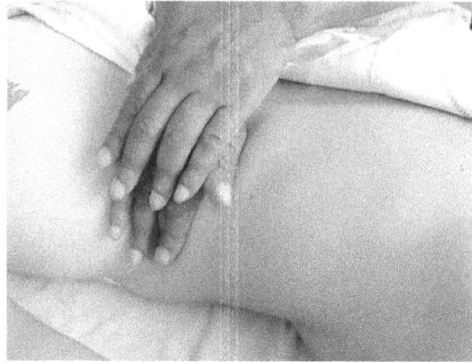

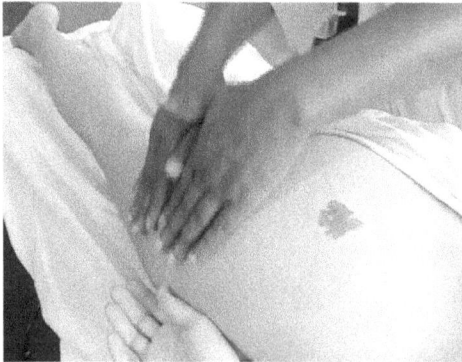

Deep circles on spine from coccyx to 7th cervical, push down spine, vibrate up spine. Effleurage. Instruct client to turn towards therapist, onto back.

Abdominal technique with deep breathing. Autogenic breathing exercises. Neck roll and pull. Effleurage chest, chin, cheeks and forehead.

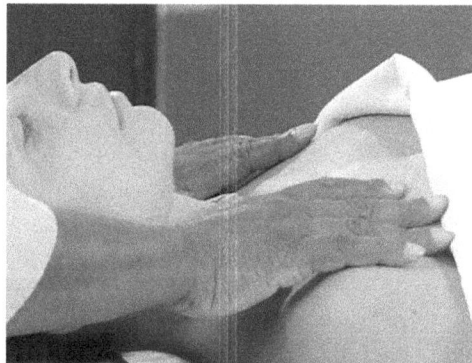

LYMPHATIC MASSAGE PROCEDURE

1. GROUND
2. CIRCLE SHOULDERS - 3 CIRCLES - L-R, 3X
3. EFFLURAGE - 3X BELOW CLAVICLE
4. THUMB CIRCLES STERNAL NOTCH
5. THUMB CIRCLES – BASE OF NECK ANTERIOR TO POSTERIOR & BACK
6. THUMB CIRCLES BEHIND CLAVICLE MED – LATERAL TO ACROM.
7. THUMB CIRCLES OVER TRAPS FROM BASE OF NECK TO ACROM
8. PIVOT THUMBS TO OCCIPITAL RIDGE – DOWN NECK WITH CRESCENTS
9. OPENING - 4 FLAT FINGERS - SLIDE ALONG TRAPS TO EDGE OF SHOULDER
10. PULL AND RELEASE TRAPS - 3X
11. HAVE CLIENT ARCH BACK, FINGER CIRCLES (TOWARDS SPINE) – UP, UP, UP ALONG SPINE - WAIST TO SHOULDERS
12. ROLL SHOULDERS - 6X – PUMP 3X
13. THUMB CIRCLES – STERNAL NOTCH – 3X
14. THUMB CIRCLES UNDER CHIN – 3X
15. FINGER CIRCLES – MID PT CHIN – UNDER LOWER MAND TO EAR
16. FINGER CIRCLES DOWN NECK
17. FINGER CIRCLES UNDER MANDIBLE TO ANGLE OF JAW
18. FLAT FINGER CIRCLES UP TO TEMPLE
19. FEEL FOR ENERGY AT CORNER OF EYE
20. FLAT FINGERS – TOP OF CHIN – CIRCLE TO ANGLE OF JAW – UP TO TEMPLE
21. TOP LIP – CIRCLE IN TOWARDS CENTER
22. CHANGE DIR DOWN SIDE OF MOUTH TO CHIN – TO ANGLE OF JAW – UP TO TEMPLE
23. UNDER EYES – THUMB CIRCLES – PULL BACK
24. STROKE GABELLA
25. 2 FINGERS TOP AND SIDE OF NOSE – DOWN, BACK TO BRIDGE
26. FLATTEN AT CORNER OF NOSE – FINGER CIRCLES DOWN TO SIDE OF MOUTH AND THEN UP TO TEMPLE
27. THUMB CIRCLES UNDER EYES – PULL BACK
28. STROKE GABELLA – WRINKLE RIGHT EYEBROW
29. STROKE GABELLA - WRINKLE LEFT EYEBROW

30. STROKE GABELLA - FINGER CIRCLES UNDER EYEBROWS – MED TO LATERAL
31. THUMB CIRCLES UNDER EYE – PULL BACK
32. STROKE GABELLA – WRINKLE BOTH EYEBROWS AT SAME TIME
33. THUMB CIRCLES UNDER EYE - PULL BACK
34. 6 CIRCLES INSIDE CORNER OF EYE
35. (Rt side of table) HAND OVER TOP OF HEAD – 2 FINGERS 3RD EYE – PRESS, PULL OVER 3RD EYE
36. (Back to top of table) - FLAT FINGERS OVER FOREHEAD – MED TO LAT – 2 SECTIONS – CIRCLE OUT
37. THUMB SLIDES OVER FOREHEAD - 3X
38. SCALP TWIST – TOO & FRO, UP & DOWN, BACK & FORTH
39. TWIST EARS – BOTTOM - UP
40. FINGER IN EARS – CIRCLE 3X TOWARDS YOU, 3X AWAY, 3X ALT, 3X TOWARDS YOU
41. PUMP TRAGER – 6X
42. PULL EARS DOWN –TOP TO BOTTOM
43. CIRCLES AT MASTOID – 6X
44. (Rt side of table) THUMB SLIDES – 3X – FOREHEAD, EYE-NOSE, NOSE - MOUTH
45. HAND TOP OF HEAD – FINGER MID CHIN – CIRCLE TO EAR
46. (Left side of table) THUMB SLIDES – 3X – FOREHEAD, EYE-NOSE, NOSE - MOUTH
47. HAND TOP OF HEAD – FINGER MID CHIN – CIRCLE TO EAR
48. CRESCENTS - SIDE OF NECK
49. THUMB TWISTS OVER CLAVICLE
50. EFFLURAGE
51. EFFLURAGE CHIN - FINGERTIPS, CHEEK - THUMB, FOREHEAD - THUMB SLIDES
52. (Move to left side of table) UNCOVER LEFT ARM
53. OPEN AXILLA, 4 FLAT FINGERS
    PRESS IN RELEASE
    PRESS IN 3 CIRCLE OUT
    PRESS IN RELEASE
    PRESS IN 3 CIRCLES IN
    PRESS IN RELEASE
    PRESS IN 3 CIRCLES OUT
54. HOLD ARM UP –SHAKE DOWN – FINGERTIPS TO SHOULDERS

55. LIE ARM DOWN – PUSH PULL – SHOULDER TO FINGERTIPS – FINGERTIPS TO SHOULDERS - 3X
56. CHOO-CHOO –SHOULDER TO FINGERTIPS – FINGERTIPS TO SHOULDERS - 2-1/2 X TO ELBOW – PLACE ELBOW IN LEFT HAND
57. FINGER CIRCLES AT ELBOW, TOP, BOTTOM, SIDES
58. CHOO-CHOO FROM ELBOW TO WRIST AND SPREAD THE HAND
59. PUMP WEBBING BETWEEN FINGERS, LITTLE TO THUMB
60. THUMB CIRCLES OVER BACK OF HAND –KNUCKLE TO WRIST IN 3 SECTION (CHICKEN FOOT)
61. MILK FINGERS, ALTERNATELY, 2 AT A TIME, MIDDLE & LITTLE, RING & INDEX, THEN THUMB
62. LIFT HAND UP – PUMP FINGERS DOWN – INDEX TO LITTLE FINGER THEN THUMB
63. DEEP CIRCLES OVER CENTER OF PALM (LAO GONG)
64. PUMP SIDES OF PALMS TO WRIST W/THUMBS
65. ROTATE WRIST – 3X L, 3X R
66. WRIST IN ARMPIT – 2 HANDED SCOOB – SHOULDER TO ELBOW - 3X
67. WRIST OUT OF ARMPIT, PLACE ON YOUR ABDOMEN - 2 HANDED SCOOB - ELBOW TO WRIST, WRIST TO ELBOW, ELBOW TO WRIST
68. TAKE CLIENT'S LEFT HAND WITH YOUR RIGHT HAND & LIFT ARM - 1 HANDED SCOOB – ELBOW TO SHOULDER – ALL 4 SIDES OF UPPER ARM – 3X
69. HOLD ARM UP – PUMP DOWN – FINGERTIPS TO SHOULDER
70. LIE ARM DOWN, EFFLURAGE – FINGERTIPS TO SHOULDER - 3X – LIGHT, SLOW
71. COVER ARM
72. UNCOVER CHEST AND ABDOMEN
73. ADDRESS LEFT BREAST – PRESSING 3X – INFERIOR TO SUPERIOR, MEDIAL TO LATERAL, DOWN - 1, 2, 3
74. FINGER CIRCLES AROUND OUTER PORTION OF BREAST, MEDIAL TO LATERAL ENDING AT AXILLA, AROUND UP TOWARDS AXILLA – REVERSE CIRCLES ON SIDE OF BREAST MOVING FLUID UP TO AXILLA, CHANGE DIRECTION AND CONTINUE BACK TO BEGINNING
75. ROTATE BREAST – UP, OVER AND RELEASE – 3X TOWARDS AXILLA, 3X TOWARDS WAIST
76. FLAT FINGER CIRCLES OVER ABDOMEN FROM RIGHT HIP TO LEFT HIP, CHANGE DIRECTION, THEN ALONG BOTTOM OF ABDOMEN BACK TO RIGHT HIP.

77. (Go to head of table) – – HANDS OVER PECS ON EITHER SIDE OF STERNUM, FLAT FINGER CIRCLES IN TOWARDS STERNUM TO ZYPHOID PROCESS – SPREAD FINGERS BETWEEN INTERCOSTAL SPACES – CIRCLE OUT LATERALLY THEN CIRCLE UP TO AXILLA
78. THUMB SLIDES OVER UPPER THORACIC - STOP AT NIPPLE LINE – BILATERALLY
79. FLAT HANDED PUMPS AT SIDE OF RIB CAGE BACK UP FROM WAIST TO AXILLA

80. COVER UP BODY – MOVE TO RIGHT SIDE OF TABLE & UNCOVER RIGHT LEG & THIGH
81. FLAT FINGER CIRCLES IN INGUNAL
82. FINGER CIRCLES (1 FINGER) OVER INGUNAL FOLD, MEDIAL TO LATERL, OUT TO TROCHANTER
83. ROCK LEG – HIP TO KNEE 4X – KNEE TO FOOT 4X – KNEE TO HIP 4X
84. SHAKE LEG – HIP TO FOOT, FOOT, FOOT TO HIP
85. PUSH-PULL – HIP TO FOOT – FOOT TO HIP
86. CHOO-CHOO – HIP TO FOOT – FOOT TO HIP
87. 2 HANDED SCOOB – HIP TO KNEE
88. T.C. AROUND KNEE
89. PALM OVER PATELLA – CIRCLE 3X RIGHT, 3X LEFT
90. 2 HANDED SCOOB DOWN TO FOOT
91. TURN – SPREAD FOOT
92. FOOT OF TABLE – PULL TOES – LITTLE TO BIG
93. SCOOB BOTTOM OF FOOT - SWITCH HANDS, SCOOB UP BACK OF LEG TO POPITEAL SPACE – FINGER CIRCLES 3X IN POPIETAL SPACE
94. T.C. – BETWEEN MEDIAL & LATERAL MALLEOLUS – MEDIAL TO LATERAL, LATERAL TO MEDIAL
95. FINGER CIRCLES BETWEEN METATARSALS – FROM BASE OF TOES TO ANKLE – 3X
96. ROTATE FOOT – 3X LEFT, 3X RIGHT
97. PUMP MED & LAT MALLEOLUS W/BASE OF PALMS 4X
98. SCOOB UP LEG TO RIGHT HIP THEN DIAGONALLY ACROSS BODY TO LEFT AXILLA.
99. COVER RIGHT LEG, UNCOVER RIGHT ARM

100. (Move to right side of table) UNCOVER RIGHT ARM
101. OPEN AXILLA, 4 FLAT FINGERS
        PRESS IN RELEASE
        PRESS IN 3 CIRCLE OUT
        PRESS IN RELEASE
        PRESS IN 3 CIRCLES IN
        PRESS IN RELEASE
        PRESS IN 3 CIRCLES OUT
102. HOLD ARM UP –SHAKE DOWN – FINGERTIPS TO SHOULDERS
103. LIE ARM DOWN – PUSH PULL – SHOULDER TO FINGERTIPS – FINGERTIPS TO SHOULDERS - 3X
104. CHOO-CHOO –SHOULDER TO FINGERTIPS – FINGERTIPS TO SHOULDERS - 2-1/2 X TO ELBOW – PLACE ELBOW IN RIGHT HAND
105. FINGER CIRCLES AT ELBOW, TOP, BOTTOM, SIDES
106. CHOO-CHOO FROM ELBOW TO WRIST AND SPREAD THE HAND
107. PUMP WEBBING BETWEEN FINGERS, LITTLE TO THUMB
108. THUMB CIRCLES OVER BACK OF HAND –KNUCKLE TO WRIST IN 3 SECTION (CHICKEN FOOT)
109. MILK FINGERS, ALTERNATELY, 2 AT A TIME, MIDDLE & LITTLE, RING & INDEX, THEN THUMB
110. LIFT HAND UP – PUMP FINGERS DOWN – INDEX TO LITTLE FINGER THEN THUMB
111. DEEP CIRCLES OVER CENTER OF PALM (LAO GONG)
112. PUMP SIDES OF PALMS TO WRIST W/THUMBS
113. ROTATE WRIST – 3X L, 3X R
114. WRIST IN ARMPIT – 2 HANDED SCOOB – SHOULDER TO ELBOW - 3X
115. WRIST OUT OF ARMPIT, PLACE ON YOUR ABDOMEN - 2 HANDED SCOOB - ELBOW TO WRIST, WRIST TO ELBOW, ELBOW TO WRIST
116. TAKE CLIENT'S LEFT HAND WITH YOUR RIGHT HAND & LIFT ARM - 1 HANDED SCOOB – ELBOW TO SHOULDER – ALL 4 SIDES OF UPPER ARM – 3X
117. HOLD ARM UP – PUMP DOWN – FINGERTIPS TO SHOULDER
118. LIE ARM DOWN, EFFLURAGE – FINGERTIPS TO SHOULDER - 3X – LIGHT, SLOW
119. COVER ARM

120. COVER UP ARM AND UNCOVER THORACIC & ABDOMEN

121. (Go to head of table) – HANDS OVER PECS ON EITHER SIDE OF STERNUM, FLAT FINGER CIRCLES IN TOWARDS STERNUM TO ZYPHOID PROCESS – SPREAD FINGERS BETWEEN INTERCOSTAL SPACES – CIRCLE OUT LATERALLY THEN CIRCLE UP TO AXILLA
122. THUMB SLIDES OVER UPPER THORACIC - STOP AT NIPPLE LINE – BILATERALLY
123. FLAT HANDED PUMPS AT SIDE OF RIB CAGE BACK UP FROM WAIST TO AXILLA
124. (Move to right side of table) ADDRESS RIGHT BREAST – PRESSING 3X – INFERIOR TO SUPERIOR – MEDIAL TO LATERAL – DOWN, 1,2,3
125. FINGER CIRCLES AROUND OUTER PORTION OF BREAST, MEDIAL TO LATERAL ENDING AT AXILLA, AROUND UP TOWARDS ARMPIT – REVERSE CIRCLES ON SIDE OF BREAST MOVING FLUID UP TO AXILLA, CHANGE DIRECTION AND CONTINUE BACK TO BEGINNING
126. ROTATE BREAST – UP, OVER AND RELEASE – 3X TOWARDS AXILLA, 3X TOWARDS WAIST
127. FLAT FINGER CIRCLES DIAGONALLY FROM RIGHT AXILLA TO LEFT HIP
128. REVERSE FINGER CIRCLES OVER ABDOMEN FROM LEFT HIP TO RIGHT HIP, CHANGE DIRECTION, THEN ALONG BOTTOM OF ABDOMEN BACK TO LEFT HIP
129. COVER UP BODY.
130. (Move to left side of table) - UNCOVER LEFT LEG & THIGH
131. FLAT FINGER CIRCLES IN INGUNAL
132. FINGER CIRCLES (1 FINGER) OVER INGUNAL FOLD, MEDIAL TO LATERL, OUT TO TROCHANTER
133. ROCK LEG – HIP TO KNEE 4X – KNEE TO FOOT 4X – KNEE TO HIP 4X
134. SHAKE LEG – HIP TO FOOT, FOOT, FOOT TO HIP
135. PUSH-PULL – HIP TO FOOT – FOOT TO HIP
136. CHOO-CHOO – HIP TO FOOT – FOOT TO HIP
137. 2 HANDED SCOOB – HIP TO KNEE
138. T.C. AROUND KNEE
139. PALM OVER PATELLA – CIRCLE 3X RIGHT, 3X LEFT
140. 2 HANDED SCOOB DOWN TO FOOT

141. TURN – SPREAD FOOT
142. FOOT OF TABLE – PULL TOES – LITTLE TO BIG
143. SCOOB BOTTOM OF FOOT - SWITCH HANDS, SCOOB UP BACK OF LEG TO POPITEAL SPACE – FINGER CIRCLES 3X IN POPIETAL SPACE
144. T.C. – BETWEEN MEDIAL & LATERAL MALLEOLUS – MEDIAL TO LATERAL, LATERAL TO MEDIAL
145. FINGER CIRCLES BETWEEN METATARSALS – FROM BASE OF TOES TO ANKLE – 3X
146. ROTATE FOOT – 3X LEFT, 3X RIGHT
147. PUMP MED & LAT MALLEOLUS W/BASE OF PALMS 4X
148. SCOOB UP LEG TO LEFT HIP THEN DIAGONALLY ACROSS BODY TO RIGHT AXILLA
149. UNCOVER RIGHT LEG (DO NOT COVER UP LEFT LEG), ASK CLIENT TO BEND KNEES, DRAPE SHEET BETWEEN LEGS, LOCK FEET.
150. MOVE TO LEFT SIDE OF TABLE
151. SHAKE LEFT LEG – ANKLE TO KNEE – TOP & BOTTOM, SHAKE UP SIDES
152. PAT UP – ANKLE TO KNEE 3X
153. 2 HANDED SCOOB (TOP OPEN, BOTTOM CLOSED) – ANKLE TO KNEE
154. CIRCLES OVER PATELLA/POPITEAL 3X LEFT, 3X RIGHT
155. PUMP PATELLA 3X
156. SHAKE DOWN THIGH – TOP & BOTTOM/SIDES – KNEE TO HIP
157. PAT HAMS – KNEE TO HIP 3X
158. SCOOB DOWN (BOTTOM OPEN, TOP CLOSED) – KNEE TO HIP
159. FINGER CIRCLES ALONG GLUTEAL & INGUNAL FOLD – MEDIAL TO LATERAL – MEETING AT TROCHANTER
160. MOVE TO RIGHT SIDE OF TABLE – **RIGHT LEG SAME AS LEFT LEG**
161. FOLD SHEET DOWN TO WAIST & MAKE DIAPER
162. DEEP FLAT FINGER CIRCLES OVER ABDOMEN FROM LEFT SIDE –WORKING UNDER ABDOMEN TO RIGHT SIDE AND THEN FROM RIGHT HIP OVER ABDOMEN TO LEFT HIP
163. DIAMOND SHAPED EFFLURAGE, UNDER RIBS AND OVER ABDOMEN

164. UNLOCK FEET AND EXTEND LEGS
165. THUMB OVER THUMB ON INSIDE OF RIGHT LEG – FROM ANKLE TO INNER THIGH
166. WAVE FROM ANKLE TO HIP AND THEN DIAGONALLY ACROSS THE BODY TO THE LEFT AXILLA
167. THUMB SLIDES ACROSS LEFT SIDE OF LEG AND TORSO – MEDIAL TO LATERAL FROM ANKLE TO AXILLA – LATERAL SIDE OF LEG
168. WAVE UP LEFT LEG TO AXILLA – CIRCLE 3X
169. MOVE TO OTHER SIDE OF TABLE AND REPEAT ON OPPOSITE SIDE
170. EFFLURAGE –   LEFT SIDE, ANKLE TO AXILLA
         LEFT ARM, FINGERTIPS TO SHOULDERS
         RIGHT SIDE, ANKLE TO AXILLA
         RIGHT ARM, FINGERTIPS TO SHOULDERS
         BOTH LEGS, TORSO, ANKLE TO AXILLA
         BOTH HANDS, ARMS & SHOULDER
         CIRCLE AROUND EARS – TOWARDS YOU

171. COVER CLIENT UP – FRONT OF BODY DONE.

172. HAVE CLIENT TURN OVER – AWAY FROM YOU ONTO STOMACH, MOVE TO HEAD OF TABLE
173. SCALP TWISTS – 3 DIRECTIONS
174. CRANIO COMPRESSIONS - TEMPORALIS, PARIETAL, OCCUPITAL (6 SEC. EACH)
175. CURL FINGERS AT OCCIPITAL RIDGE AND OCCIPITAL VIBRATION
176. MOVE TO SIDE OF TABLE – SCOOB & PULL (DOWN) NECK
177. POP BACK OF NECK - PULL SKIN UP
178. MOVE BACK TO HEAD OF TABLE
179. FINGER CIRCLES ALONG SIDE OF CRANIUM – TEMPORALIS, PARIETAL, OCCIPITAL TO MASTOID
180. MOHAWK - 6 SEC EACH – FRONTALIS TO OCCIPUT
181. MOVE TO SIDE OF TABLE – TRAP TWISTS – BI-LATERAL (HOOK AND SPADE OVER TRAPS), END WITH 3 PUMPS
182. MOVE TO HEAD OF TABLE – UNCOVER BACK

183. FLAT HAND CIRCLES TOWARDS SPINE DOWN BACK – SHOULDERS TO WAIST
184. SPREAD FINGERS – FINGER CIRCLES BETWEEN INTERCOSTAL & CIRCLE BACK UP TO AXILLA
185. THUMBS AT BASE OF NECK – TOP OF TRAPS, FINGER CIRCLES OUT TO ACROMION PROCESS.
186. MOVE TO RIGHT SIDE OF TABLE – MONKEY CLIMB – 3 SECTIONS – INFERIOR TO SUPERIOR, WAIST TO SHOULDER, LATERAL TO MEDIAL
187. **REPEAT ON OTHER SIDE**
188. MONKEY CLIMB UP SPINE FROM WAIST TO SHOULDER (UP ALONG SPINE)
189. THUMB SLIDES OVER KIDNEYS - ALTERNATE & PARALLEL – 3X EACH SIDE, THEN PUMP KIDNEYS 3X
190. INCH WORM UP BACK – PALMS UP, FINGERS FORWARD, THUMB & PALMS DOWN – TO SHOULDERS
191. COVER BODY, MOVE TO LEFT SIDE OF TABLE, UNCOVER LEFT LEG & GLUTE
192. ADDRESS GLUTEAL – DOWN 1,2,3 N-S, E-W
193. KNEAD GLUTE (CRESCENTS) – SUPERIOR TO INFERIOR, INFERIOR TO SUPERIOR
194. FULLING – PULL ON SKIN QUICKLY (SMALL LIGHT PINCHES) – SUPERIOR TO INFERIOR, LATERAL TO MEDIAL, INFERIOR TO SUPERIOR, MEDIAL TO LATERAL
195. FLAT FINGER CIRCLES OVER SIDE OF GLUTEAL – 3 AT TOP MEDIAL TO LATERAL – 1 AT BASE
196. PLACE HAND OVER KIDNEY – OTHER HAND WORKS GLUTEAL FOLD TO HIP – MEDIAL TO LATERAL – CIRCLES 1,2,3
197. SHAKE LEG – HIP TO ANKLE – ANKLE TO HIP
198. PUSH PULL – HIP TO ANKLE – ANKLE TO HIP
199. CHOO-CHOO – HIP TO ANKLE – ANKLE TO HIP
200. 2 HANDED SCOOB – HIP TO KNEE – STOP AT POPITEAL SPACE FLAT FINGER CIRCLES– CIRCLE IN – CIRCLE AROUND POPITEAL SPACE
201. SCOOB DOWN TO ANKLE
202. TURN AROUND – BEND KNEE

203. PLACE INDEX FINGERS AT BASE OF TOES – ROTATE 3X LEFT, 3X RIGHT
204. THUMB OVER THUMB – FROM BASE OF LITTLE TOE TO BIG TOE, BIG TOE TO LITTLE TOE
205. PUMP TOES DOWN TO FOOT, SMALL TO BIG.
206. PUMP DOWN SIDES, MED, CENTER, CIRCLE AROUND HEEL – PUMP HEEL
207. STROKE ACHILLES TENDON
208. THUMB ACROSS ACHILLES – SLIDE DOWN TO POPITEAL SPACE
209. CIRCLE OVER INSTEP – FLAT FINGERS
210. LAY FOOT DOWN – CURLED FINGERS – PUMP MALLEOLUS SUPERIOR DIRECTION – 3X
211. SCOOB FOOT – 3X
212. SCOOB UP BODY TO AXILLA & SCAP & PUMP 3X (VERTICAL & HORIZONTAL AT SAME TIME)
213. COVER UP – MOVE TO OTHER SIDE OF TABLE – **REPEAT FROM GLUTES TO SCOOB UP BODY**
214. COVER UP – UNCOVER OPPOSITE SIDE OF BODY – HOLD, SLIDE, TUCK
215. THUMB SLIDES – ANKLE TO AXILLA
216. KIDNEY PUMPS – 12X
217. THUMB SLIDES – WAIST TO AXILLA – CIRCLE 3X
218. WAVE ANKLE TO AXILLA
219. COVER UP – MOVE TO OPPOSITE SIDE OF TABLE – **REPEAT FROM TUCK & SLIDE**
220. UNCOVER OTHER SIDE (DO NOT COVER SIDE YOU JUST WORKED) & FOLD SHEET DOWN OVER GLUTES
221. FLAT FINGER CIRCLES OVER SPINE – LUMBAR TO CERVICAL
222. DECENDING PRESSURE POINTS ALONG SIDE OF SPINE W/PALM TWISTS, MEDIAL TO LATERAL
223. VIBRATION OVER SPINE (W/BACK OF PALM) – LUMBER TO CERVICAL
224. EFFLURAGE RIGHT SIDE, ANKLE TO AXILLA
225. EFFLURAGE RIGHT ARM, FINGERTIPS TO SHOULDER
226. EFFLURAGE LEFT ARM, ANKLE TO AXILLA
227. EFFLURAGE LEFT SIDE, FINGERTIPS TO SHOULDER
228. EFFLURAGE ANKLE TO AXILLA (BOTH SIDES SAME TIME)

229. EFFLURAGE 3X OVER WAIST/KIDNEYS, 1 STROKE UP CENTER OF BACK, UP SIDES OF BACK, SIDE OF SIDE, WAIST TO AXILLA
230. EFFLURAGE – HANDS, ARMS, SHOULDERS, CIRCLE AROUND EARS
231. COVER UP – TURN OVER
232. ROCKING – HOLD HEELS – CIRCLES IN – 30X – TRY TO GET FLUID RHYTHM OF CLIENT
233. HAVE CLIENT TAKE 3 DEEP BREATHS INTO THE ABDOMEN, PALMS OVER ABDOMEN, FOLLOW DOWN WITH INHALE, HOLD WITH EXHALE
234. 7 DEEP CIRCLES OVER ABDOMEN, CIRCLE UP WITH EACH CIRCLE (MODULATE) TO PASSIVE TOUCH, RELEASE
235. HAVE CLIENT TAKE DEEP BREATH, TENSE ALL MUSCLES AND THEN RELEASE – 3X
236. MOVE TO HEAD OF TABLE – ROLL NECK – 3X
237. EFFLURAGE BELOW CLAVICLE – 3X
238. CHIN, CHEEKS, FOREHEAD.

LYMPHGEFÄSSE
nach Sappey, Paris 1872.

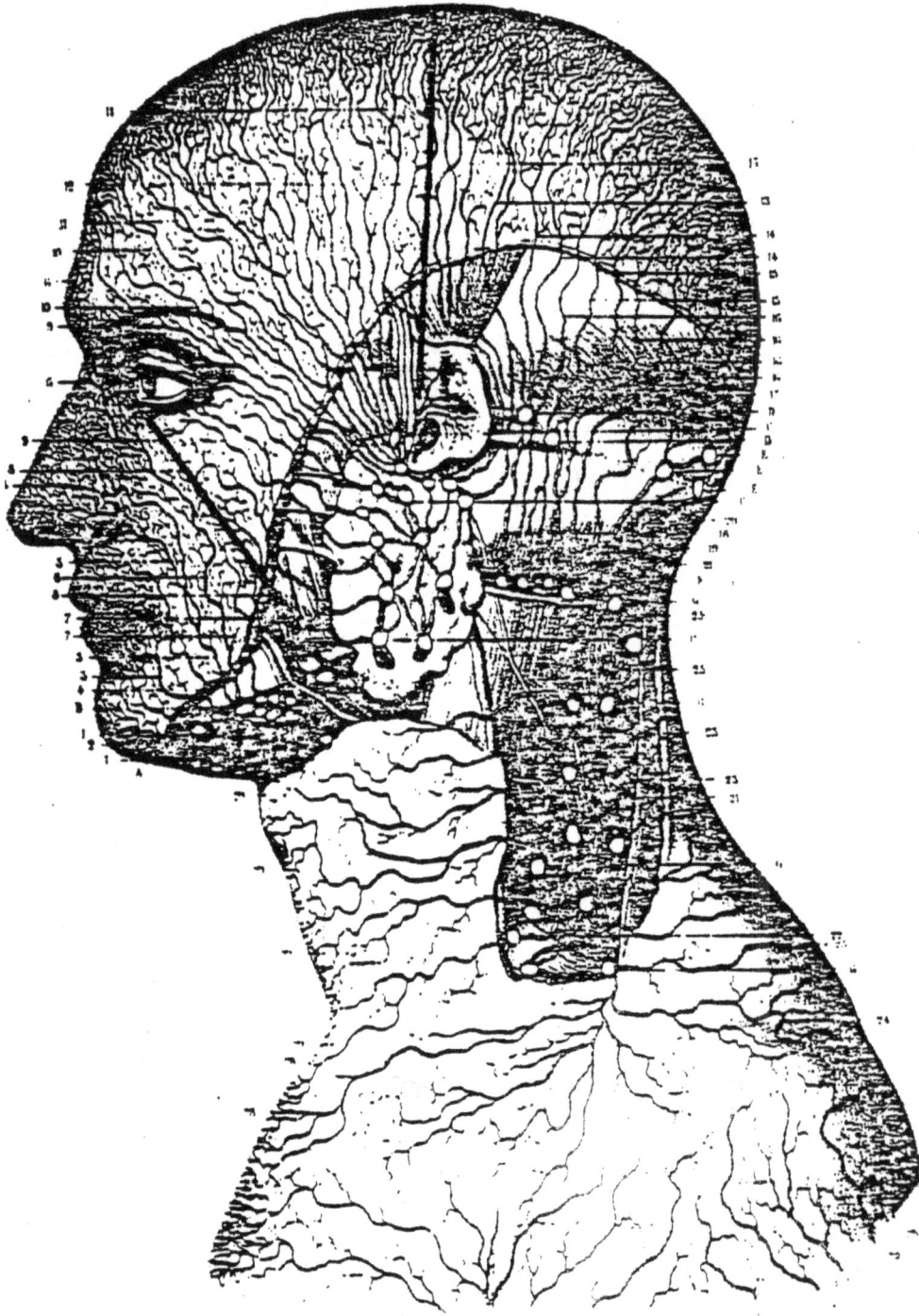

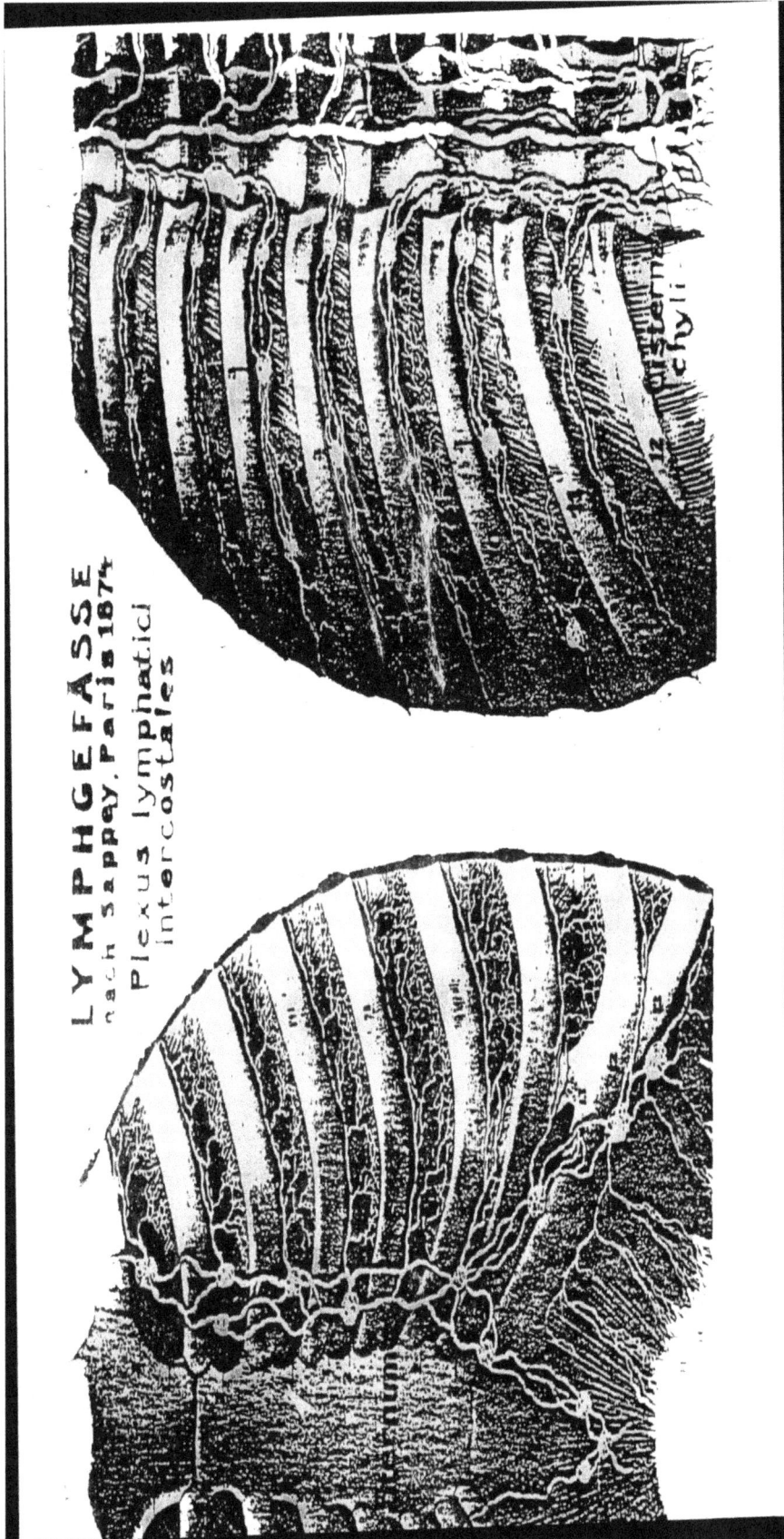

LYMPHGEFÄSSE
nach Sappey, Paris 1874

Plexus lymphatici
intercostales

cisterna
chyli

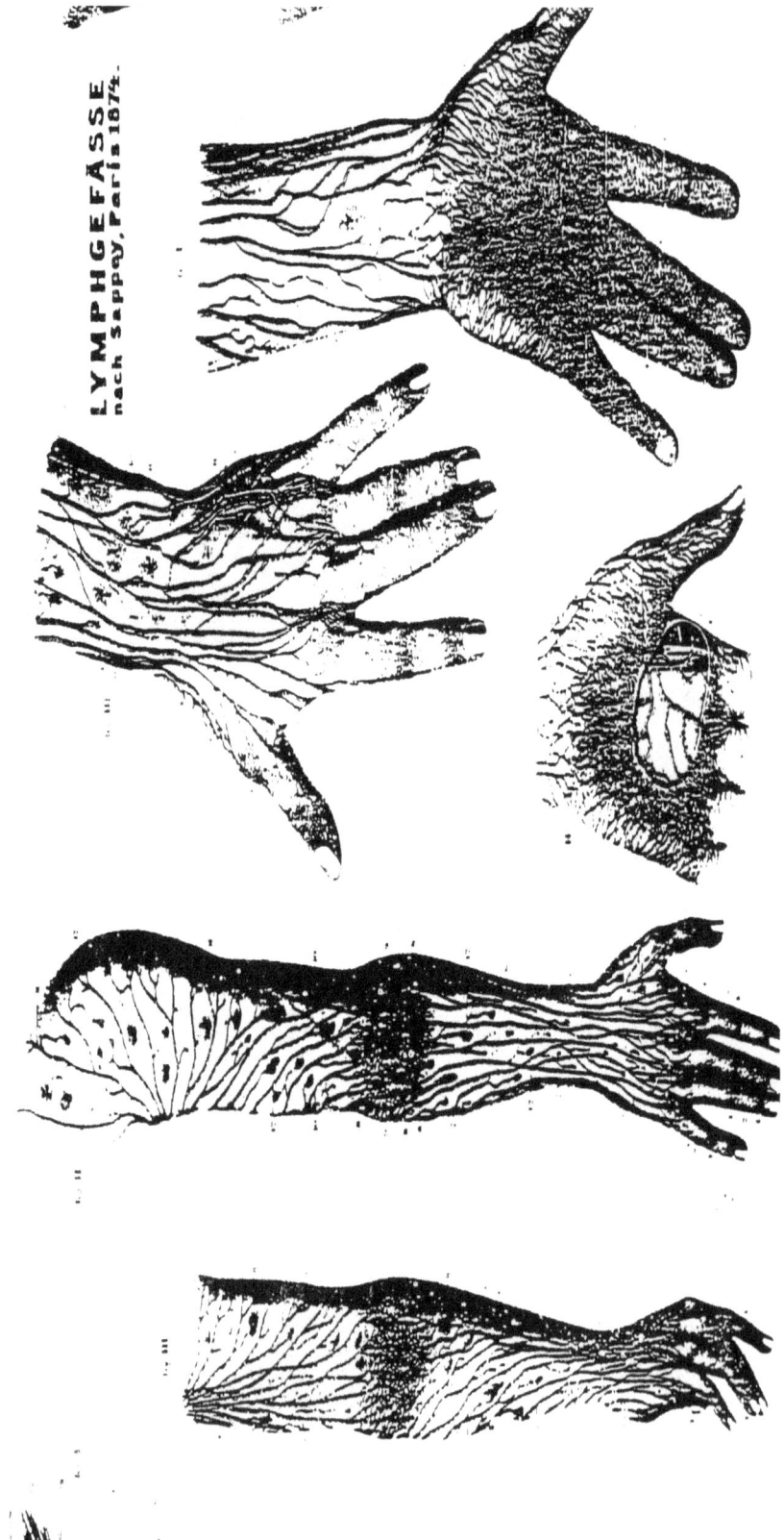

LYMPHGEFÄSSE
nach Sappy, Paris 1874.

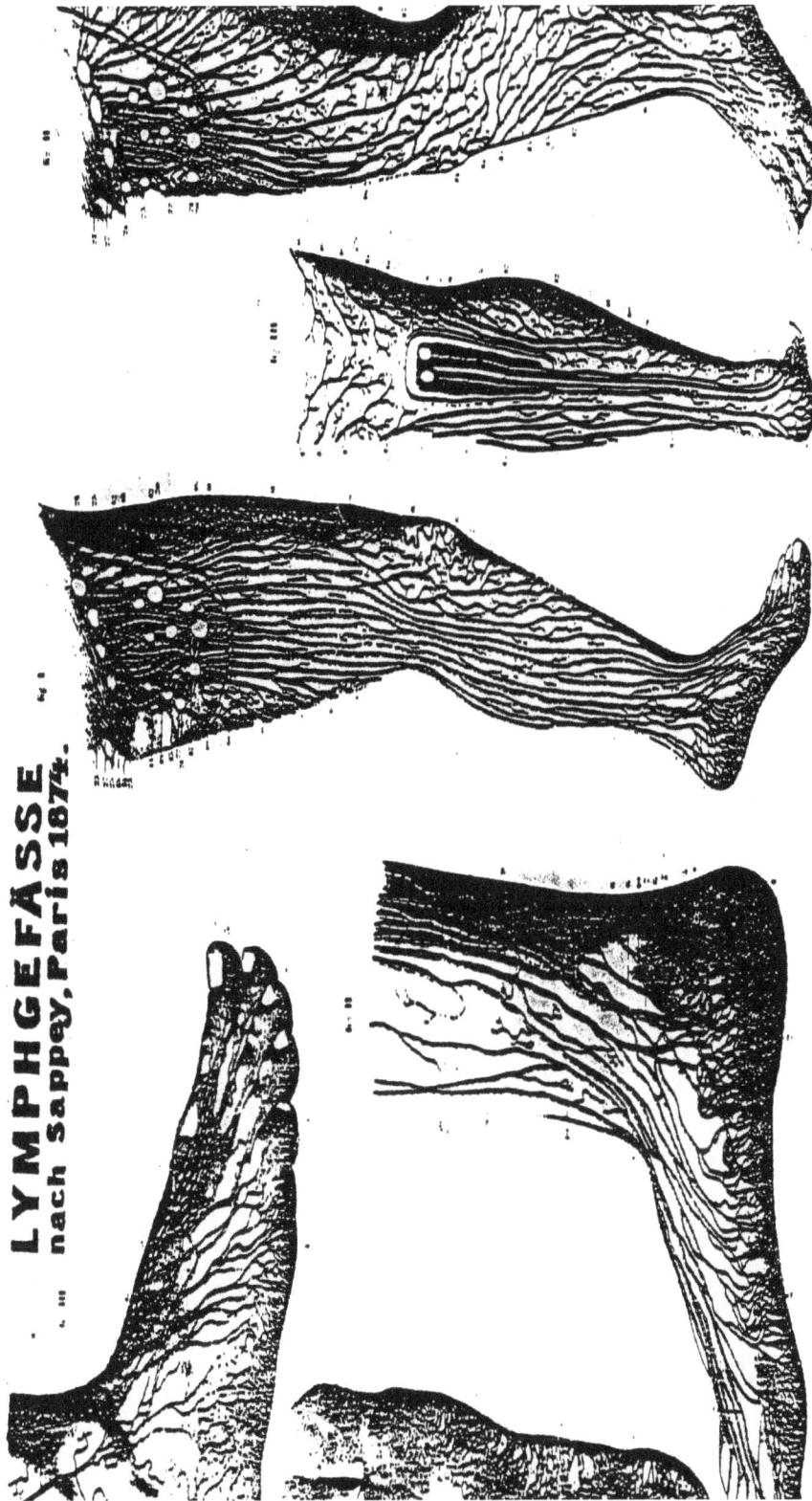

LYMPHGEFÄSSE
nach Sappey, Paris 1874.

The Lymphatic Electro-magnetic wireless circuits

ELECTRO-MAGNETIC CURRENTS AND THEIR
PROPER ANATOMICAL RELATIONS ANTERIOR
AND POSTERIOR VIEW OF OVERALL SWEEP
PLUS POLARITY CENTERS.

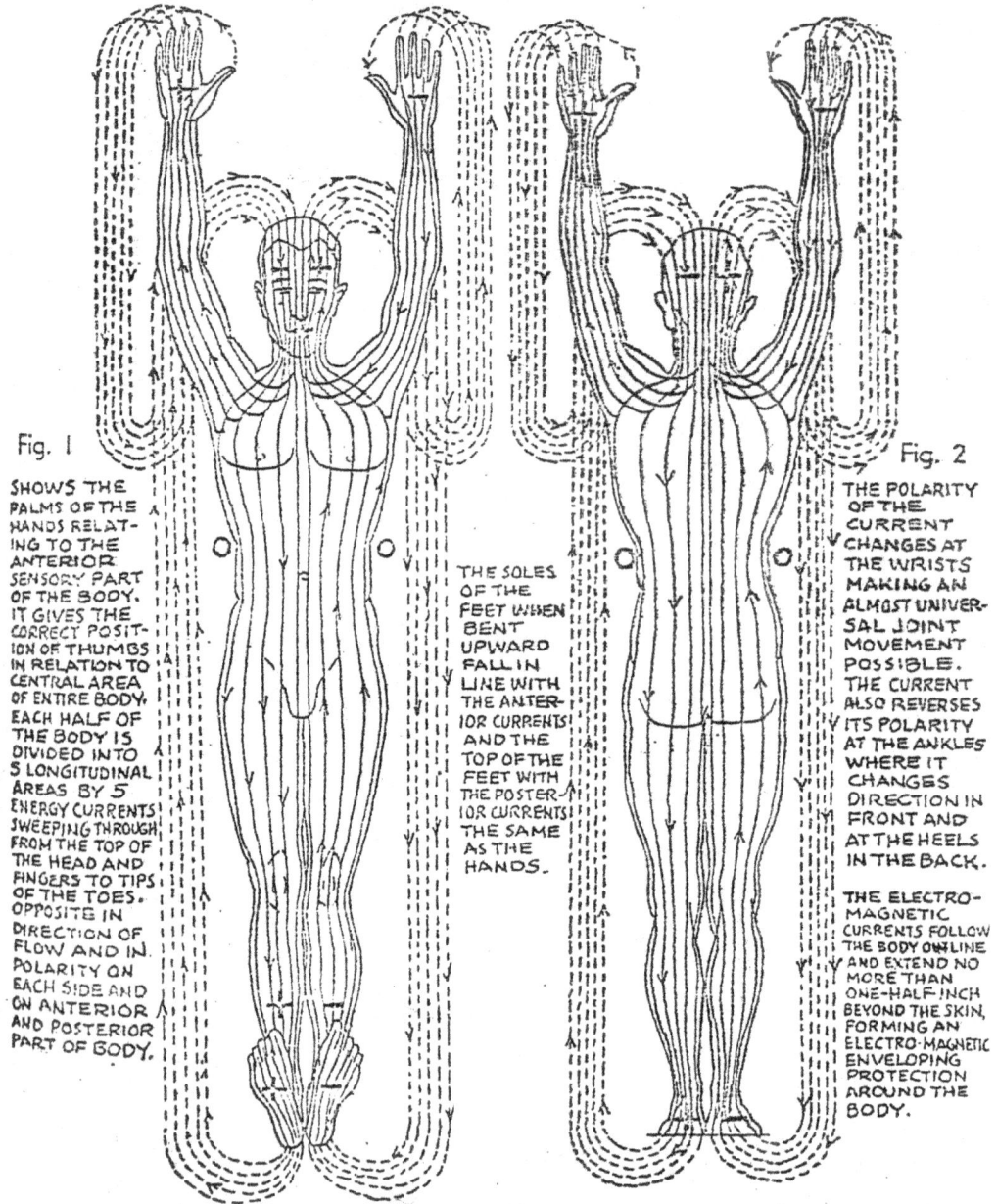

Fig. 1

SHOWS THE
PALMS OF THE
HANDS RELAT-
ING TO THE
ANTERIOR
SENSORY PART
OF THE BODY.
IT GIVES THE
CORRECT POSIT-
ION OF THUMBS
IN RELATION TO
CENTRAL AREA
OF ENTIRE BODY.
EACH HALF OF
THE BODY IS
DIVIDED INTO
5 LONGITUDINAL
AREAS BY 5
ENERGY CURRENTS
SWEEPING THROUGH
FROM THE TOP OF
THE HEAD AND
FINGERS TO TIPS
OF THE TOES.
OPPOSITE IN
DIRECTION OF
FLOW AND IN.
POLARITY ON
EACH SIDE AND
ON ANTERIOR
AND POSTERIOR
PART OF BODY.

THE SOLES
OF THE
FEET WHEN
BENT
UPWARD
FALL IN
LINE WITH
THE ANTER-
IOR CURRENTS
AND THE
TOP OF THE
FEET WITH
THE POSTER-
IOR CURRENTS
THE SAME
AS THE
HANDS.

Fig. 2

THE POLARITY
OF THE
CURRENT
CHANGES AT
THE WRISTS
MAKING AN
ALMOST UNIVER-
SAL JOINT
MOVEMENT
POSSIBLE.
THE CURRENT
ALSO REVERSES
ITS POLARITY
AT THE ANKLES
WHERE IT
CHANGES
DIRECTION IN
FRONT AND
AT THE HEELS
IN THE BACK.

THE ELECTRO-
MAGNETIC
CURRENTS FOLLOW
THE BODY OUTLINE
AND EXTEND NO
MORE THAN
ONE-HALF INCH
BEYOND THE SKIN,
FORMING AN
ELECTRO-MAGNETIC
ENVELOPING
PROTECTION
AROUND THE
BODY.

ADVANCED LYMPHATIC PROTOCOLS

The Advanced Lymphatic Protocols (ALP) are defined by the five (5) pointed star (See Fig. 1). Each point of the star represents a specific lymph gate when opened in proper sequence enhances and accelerates the flow of the lymphatic system. These gates along with the proper lymphatic pumping to detoxify thru the kidneys facilitates and increases the flow of the lymph stream and supports a gentle yet through detoxification. Without the proper sequential opening of the lymph gates combined with the detox pump even though the lymph system may be stimulated, the flow of the lymph stream will not be increased beyond aerobic activity at 15-20 liters of lymph in one hour. However, with the Advanced Lymphatic Protocols the rate of the flow of the lymph may be increased to 40 to 50 liters of lymph in one hour with no signs of toxic letheragy. By using "ALP" in partial lymphatic treatments the flow of the lymphatic system will be increased dramatically. For those whose practice of lymph drainage is limited to drainage of parts of the body rather than a whole body treatment ALP, as taught at the Foundation for Holistic Health Therapy, will improve the effectiveness of your work, i.e.; faster, longer lasting results. ALP is the lost knowledge of how to treat the lymphatic system, now re-discovered and made available to all of us who practice lymphatic drainage/massage.

THE LYMPHATIC THERAPY CHART OF THE FIVE POINTED STAR

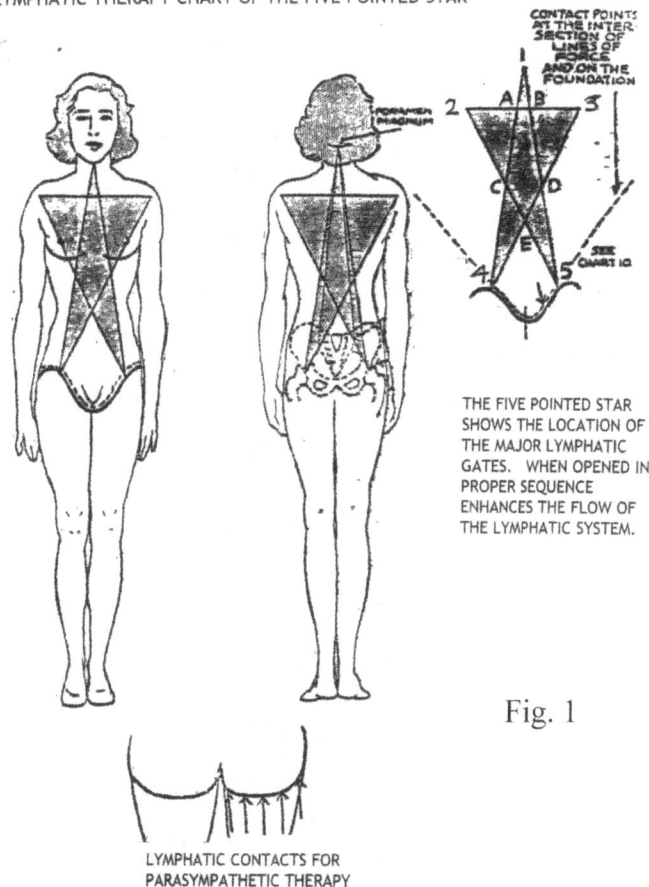

CONTACT POINTS AT THE INTERSECTION OF LINES OF FORCE AND/ON THE FOUNDATION

THE FIVE POINTED STAR SHOWS THE LOCATION OF THE MAJOR LYMPHATIC GATES. WHEN OPENED IN PROPER SEQUENCE ENHANCES THE FLOW OF THE LYMPHATIC SYSTEM.

Fig. 1

LYMPHATIC CONTACTS FOR PARASYMPATHETIC THERAPY

GLOSSARY OF TERMS

Push-pull
A two handed palmer movement, palms facing each other, moving the skin in opposite directions, from distal to proximal on the extremities.

Monkey Climbing
A two handed approach to skin from the lumbar area over the latissiumus dorsi to the top of the clavicular border of the trapezius.

Scoob
A palmar hand movement with a wave-like motion utilized on the extremities to move subcutaneous tissue from distal to proximal. The scoob can be done either with one hand or two hands, backwards and forwards.

Kidney pump
A palmar hand over hand technique, one hand resting on the top of the other, utilizing a wave like motion from the fingertip to the heel of the hand while sliding laterally between the space at the top of the pelvis and the intercostal border.

Double slide thumb
A two handed technique utilizing the thumbs and the base of the thumb medially to laterally over the large round and broad surfaces of the body.

The long circle
Spiral circles starting at the sides of the base of the nose, moving towards the lower mandible, along the mandibular border to the angle of the lower mandible and proceeding to the temple, ending at the corner of the eyes.

Rotary technique
A hand technique using the palm, the base of the thumbs, alternating one in front of the other while twisting outwards towards the little fingers, while moving laterally over the large broad, and round surfaces of the body.

Choo-choo
Palmar rotary hand movements from proximal to distal and from distal to proximal along the extremities of the body.

Break hand/foot
A flexion of the carpals and metacarpals of the hand and foot, lateral to medial.

Stationary circles
Small circles exerted with fingertip circles, applied to the intercostal area of the body.

Rocking
Rotation of the lower extremities, lateral to medial; medial to lateral.

Shaking
Palmar hand movements, moving skin vertically over the extremities of the body, proximal to distal; distal to proximal.

INDICATIONS

The following is a partial list of indications for treatment with Lymphatic Massage.

Edemas

Arm edemas – after mastectomy
Leg edemas – primary and secondary
Lipoedemas
Head edemas

Traumatic Injuries

Haematomas
Sprain or strain of joint
Subluxation of joints (eg. shoulder, finger, knee)
Fractures – pre & post surgery and post casting

Sudecks Dystrophy
Scar treatment
Stripping operations
Burn scars
Amputation stump
Hallux valgus - hammer toe
Cosmetic operations
Jaw operations – teeth, etc.
Jaw operations – post restostitis
Jaw orthopaedics
Paradontosis

Rheumatism & Arthritis

Inflamatory
 - rheumatic fever, acute polyarthritis, acute joint rheumatism – NO LYMPHATIC MASSAGE CAN
BE DONE
 - Primary Chronic Polyarthritis – PCP
 - Morbus Bechterew – spondylitis ankylosis
 - infectious arthritis
Arthrosis
Polyarthrosis Deformans
Coxarthrosis
Knee arthrosis
Metatarsal, tarsal or hallux vulgar
Shoulder arthrosis
Elbow

Handjoints
Vertebral column arthrosis

Arthropathy

Gout
Psoriatic arthropathy
Allergic arthropathy

Lupus erythematosis (SLE)
Scleroderma
Fibrositis syndrome
Tendoperiostosis - eg tennis elbow
Tendovaginitis
Bursitis
Dupuytren's Contracture
Peri-arthrosis - humero scapularis
Myogelosen
Torticollis
Panniculosis
Osteoporosis

Edema in Cerebral Region

Apoplexia (stroke)
Commotro – cerebrum – concussion
Contusion
Migraine
Headache
Meniere's Disease
Hearing problems
Tennitus
Trigeminal neuralgia
Facial paralysis
Glaucoma

Multiple Sclerosis
Herpes Zoster

Lymphatic Children

Downs Syndrome children
Infantile cerebral paralysis

(Arteriosclerosis – little can be done with M.L.D.)

Claudicatio Intermittens
Arterial ulcers
Diabetes – leg ulcers – foot and toes
Venous blockage edemas
 - venous ulcers
 - eczema
 - post thrombotic vein

Chronic Inflammatory Respiratory Conditions
 - Allergic – eg. hayfever
 - Chronic colds – sinusitus – runny nose
 - Chronic tonsilitis
 - Cattarrh of eustacian tube
 - Ear infections and fluid build up in ears
 - Chronic bronchitis
 - Asthma
 - Asthmatic bronchitis
 - Pleuritis

Chronic constipation
Ulcerous colitis
Chronic pancreas insufficiency

Vegetative changes – eg. stress
Vegetative dystonia

Pregancy
Adipositas
Cellulie

Dematological Indications

Acute vulgaris
Rosacea
Acne
Eczema
Perional dermatitis
Hairloss
Lymphostatic entheropy

Retina detachment
Mumps
Parkinsons Disease

Low back problems
Dental problems

RAMACHI
OR
SELF HELP LYMPHATIC MASSAGE

When the concept of Lymphatic Massage's immune strengthening is clearly understood, the question is invariably asked.... "can I work on myself?" The answer must be couched in relative terms, related to a scientific standard of measure and a physical state of balance that few have experienced. Now we have the transmission of RamaChi, the self help method of Lymphatic Massage. While it is not as effective as a treatment from a trained practitioner, it can be very beneficial.

This method was developed by Dr. Brown and Jon Cogan, A.K.A. Rama. It is the technique of self lymphatic as taught by Dr. Anita Childs and adapted by Dr. Brown by combining it with the expression of Tai Chi as taught by Rama. RamaChi is a dynamic, synergistic acknowledgment of the symbiotic relationship of movement, breath, and opening to spirit.

The shift to the alpha brain wave state produced by the neuro-synaptic modulation of TaiChi movement, provides a moving meditation as a platform for the acceleration of the life stream through the lymphatic system. While in the meditative state, a resonance is created with the universal harmonic and a correspondence between the five elements of TaiChi and the five major gates of the lymphatic system, to accelerate the lymph flow. There are several methods of increasing the flow of the lymph stream. However, the precise methodology of the sequential opening of the five major gates has never before been combined with a method of moving the lymph stream.

Now with the development of RamaChi, we have the best available system of self help Lymphatic Massage. Ancient knowledge, experience of health enhancement and spiritual development are contained in this simple, easy to learn set of exercises which are designed to relax mentally, strengthen physically, balance internally, and accelerate the flow of spirit through the lymphatic system. You will be successful with this method, to the extent that you master the principles of meditation and harmonious body movement

The Touch That Heals

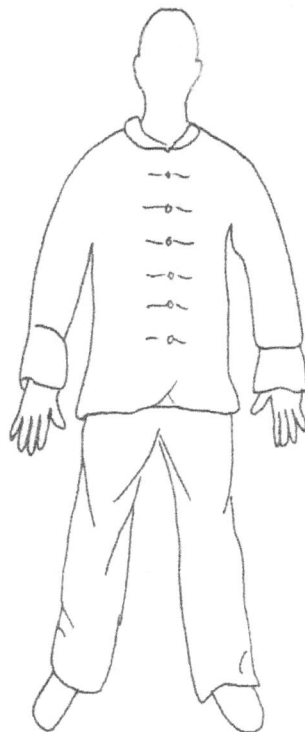

1. TAICHI BALANCE-
BREATHING-RELAXATION

2 VISUALIZE WHITE LIGHT
FLOWING DOWN FROM THE
HEART OF GOD TO YOUR
HEART AND HANDS

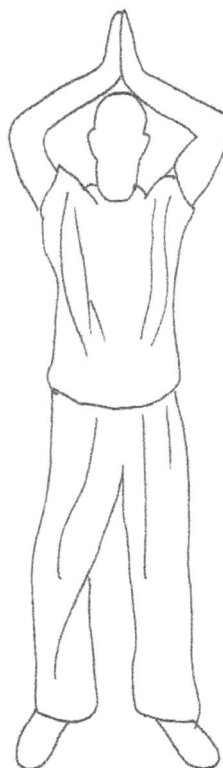

Dr. William N. Brown Ph.D., N.D., D.Sc.

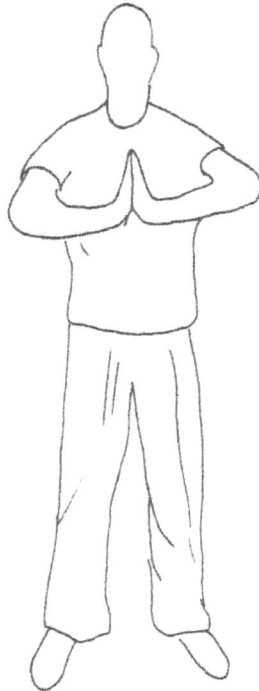

3.CONNECT WITH THE
CENTER OF THE EARTH
AND SPIRAL ENERGY UP
AROUND YOU. BREATHE IN
AND OUT RHYTHMICALLY

4. START AT MIDLINE CONTROL
POINT AND CIRCLE 3 TIMES LEFT
AND 3 TIMES RIGHT.

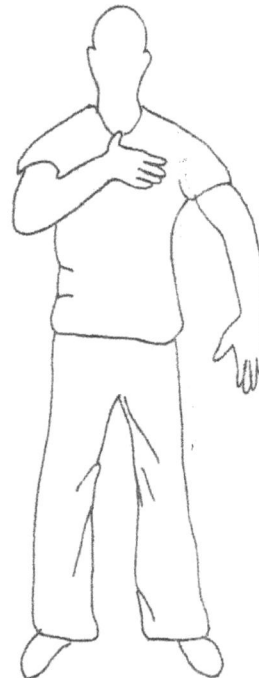

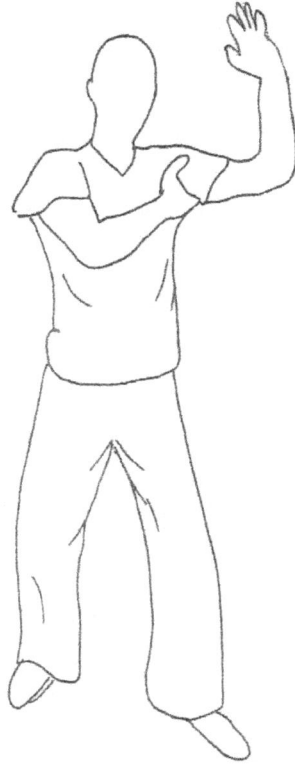

5.SPIRAL PALM OVER LEFT
ARMPIT-CIRCLE 3 TIMES LEFT
AND 3 TIMES RIGHT.

6 PUMP LYMPH IN LEFT ARM
FROM WRIST TO ELBOW.

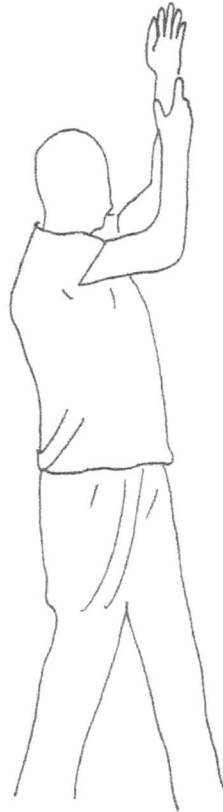

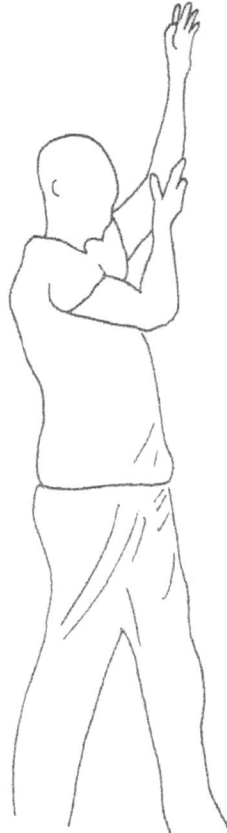

7. PUMP LYMPH IN LEFT ARM
FROM ELBOW TO ARMPIT.

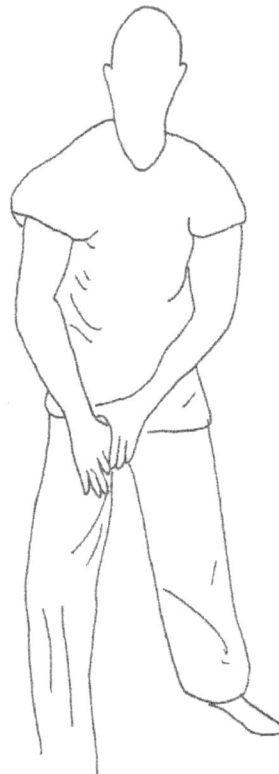

8. SPIRAL PALM OVER RIGHT INNER
THIGH-CIRCLE 3 TIMES LEFT AND 3
TIMES RIGHT.

The Touch That Heals

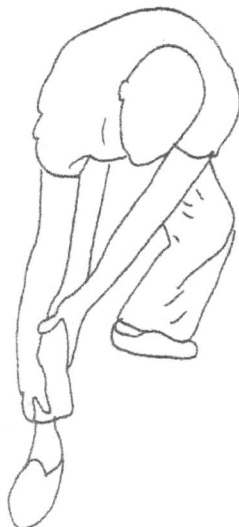

9. PUMP LYMPH IN RIGHT
LEG FROM ANKLE TO KNEE.

10. PUMP LYMPH IN RIGHT LEG
FROM KNEE TO INNER THIGH.

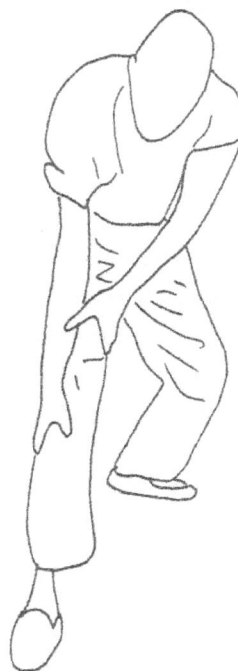

Dr. William N. Brown Ph.D., N.D., D.Sc.

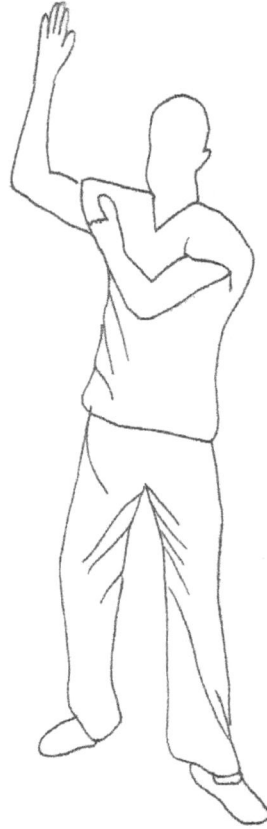

11. SPIRAL PALM OVER RIGHT
ARMPIT-CIRCLE 3 TIMES LEFT
AND 3 TIMES RIGHT.

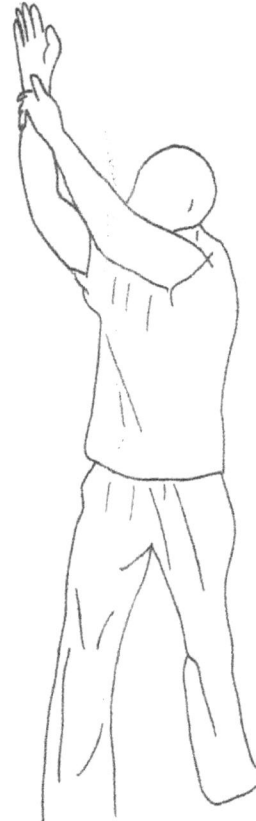

12. PUMP LYMPH IN RIGHT ARM
FROM WRIST TO ELBOW.

The Touch That Heals

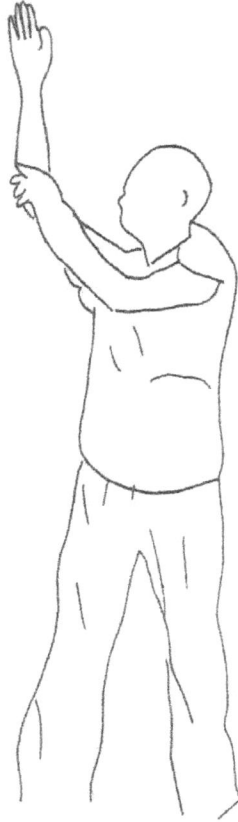

13. PUMP LYMPH IN RIGHT
ARM FROM ELBOW TO
ARMPIT.

14. SPIRAL PALM OVER LEFT
INNER THIGH-CIRCLE 3 TIMES
LEFT AND 3 TIMES RIGHT.

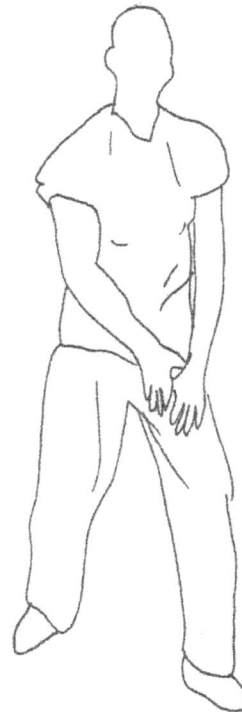

Dr. William N. Brown Ph.D., N.D., D.Sc.

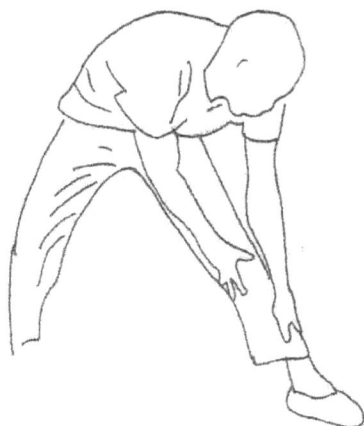

15. PUMP LYMPH IN LEFT LEG
FROM ANKLE TO KNEE.

16. PUMP LYMPH IN LEFT LEG
FROM KNEE TO INNER THIGH.

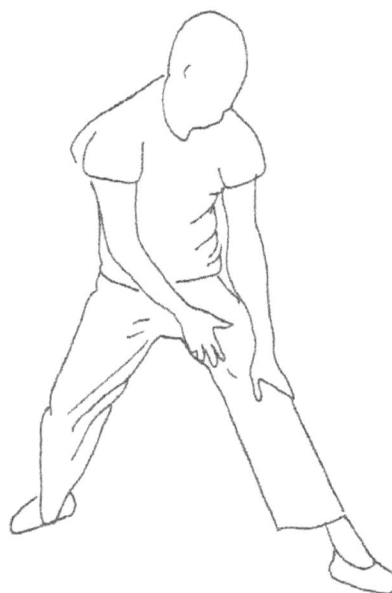

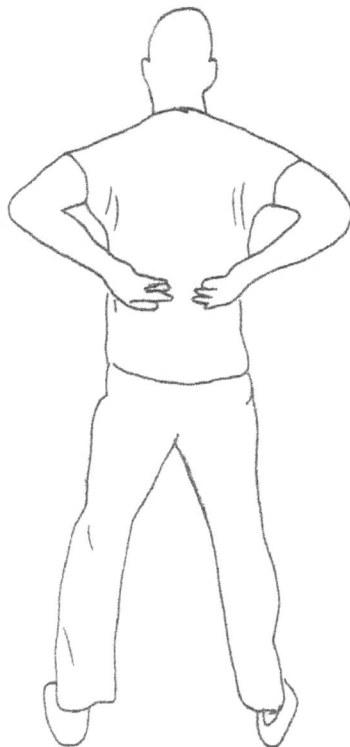

17. PUMP KIDNEYS.

18. PUMP KIDNEYS-12 TIMES.

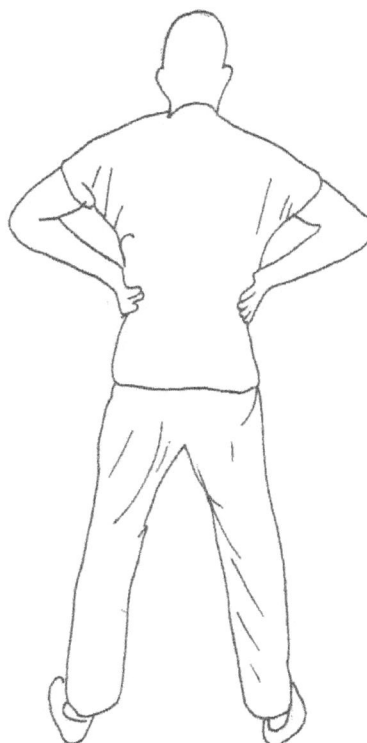

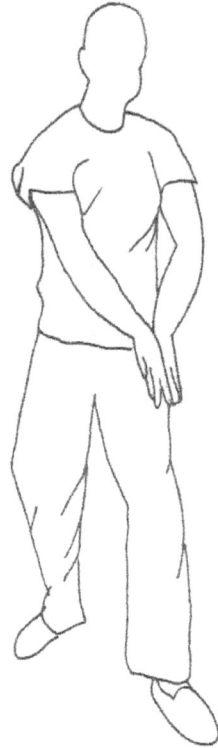

19. STAND WITH HEELS
TOGETHER. STEP OUT WITH
LEFT FOOT. PUT BACK OF
HANDS TOGETHER. WEIGHT
ON REAR LEG.

20. SHIFT WEIGHT FORWARD
AND OPEN HANDS. CONTINUE
PROCESS OF SHIFTING BACK
AND FORTH FOR 5 MINUTES
WHILE RHYTHMICALLY
BREATHING.

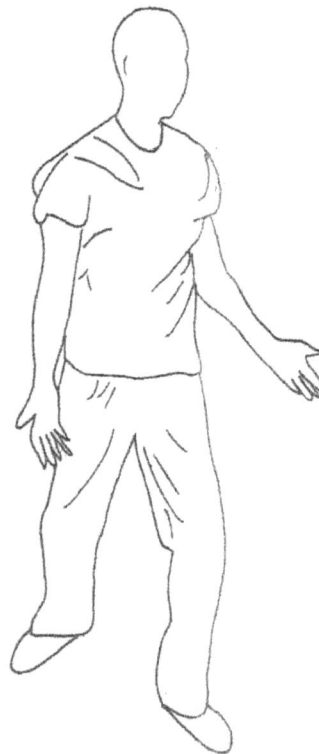

The Touch That Heals

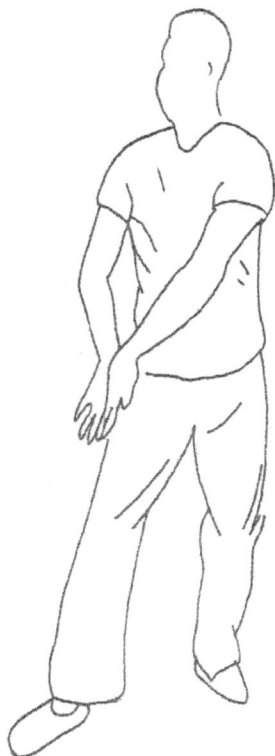

21. SLIDE LEFT FOOT BACK
AND STEP OUT WITH RIGHT
FOOT. REPEAT SHIFTING BACK
AND FORTH FOR 5 MINUTES.

22. THEN REPEAT FOR 5 MORE
MINUTES ON LEFT SIDE AND
5 MORE MINUTES ON RIGHT
SIDE.(TOTAL 20 MINUTES).

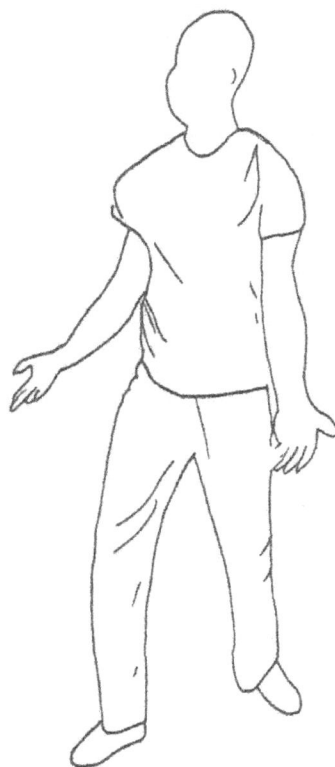

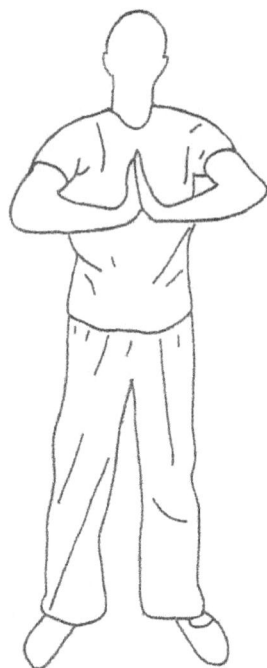

23. HEART CENTER,
GRATITUDE.

24. TAICHI BALACE-BREATHING-
RELAXATION.

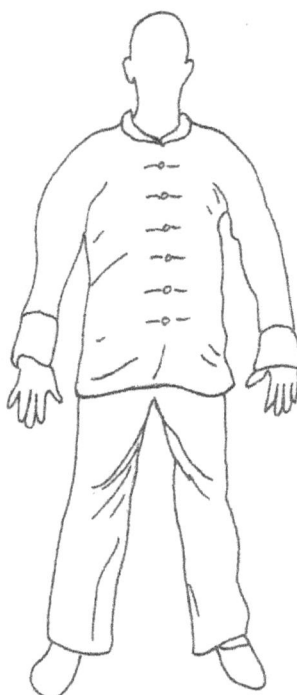

"The vibration of health resonates and embraces the mind, body and spirit."

Dr. Imhotep Aten Amenra

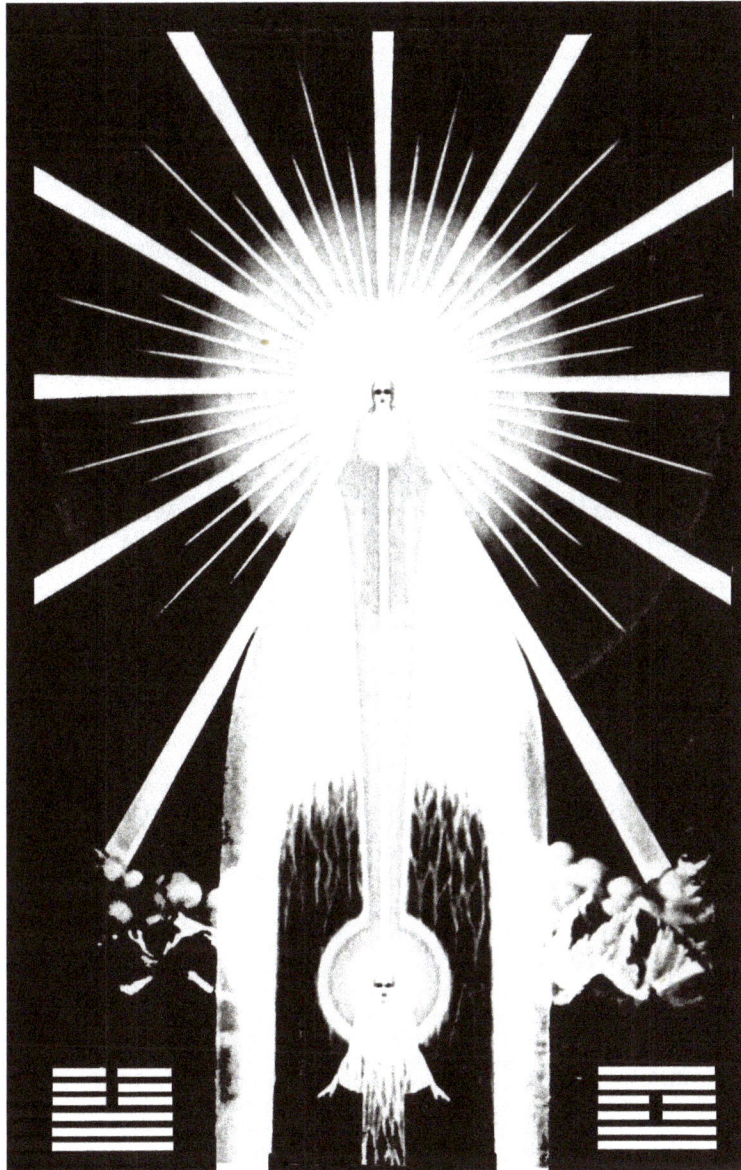

PART THREE

ANECDOTAL CASE HISTORIES

CASE # 1: MY TEACHER

I met Dr. Annie Childs in Ventura, CA in 1982. I was attending a very special school on clinical nutritional assessment. At that time, Dr. Childs was in very poor health, she could not walk across the parking lot without gasping for breath. In fact, the majority of the students in this class were in very poor health, and had come to this school to learn nutritional assessment (based on metabolic balance) as a last resort.

The course was very intensive and by lunch time most students were totally exhausted, including Dr. Childs. I took it upon myself to show the class some Tai-Chi movements in order to re-energized them. Dr. Childs was so impressed with the results of these exercises, that she offered me an exchange. If I would teach her Tai-Chi, she would teach me Lymphatic Massage. Little did I know that this exchange would change my life and restore her health.

After the three day Lymphatic Massage seminar, I worked on her almost every day for the first month, then every other day the second month. By the third month, I saw her once a week. She was now jogging four miles three times a week, swimming twice a week, teaching classes and working with clients every day! I knew then that God had blessed me with knowledge of a profound healing technique, and a good friend in Dr. Childs. However, I had yet to discover the immensity of the knowledge and skill I had gained!

In time I would learn that Lymphatic Massage was more than just a physical therapy, but a spiritual art of the highest order. Dr. Childs knew this when she taught me the white light technique which opens the doorway to the discovery of the energetic and spiritual aspect of the work. Some of us are guided by our destiny, others are dragged along by their fate. For the first time in my life, I truly felt divine guidance.

CASE #2: MY MOTHER

My mother came to see me graduate from post-graduate school and receive my Doctorate in nutrition. When she arrived, I met her at the airport. She was in a panic, "I forgot my high blood pressure medicine!" she exclaimed. As I observed her, I could see her ankles were so swollen as to resemble grapefruits and she was decidedly out of breath. I gently attempted to reassure her that everything would be alright, and thanked her for sharing my greatest academic triumph. Then I asked her, "Mom, may I take care of you for the next week?" She agreed.

The first thing I did was to give her a Lymphatic Massage. It calmed her right down and reduced the swelling in her ankles. Then I did a nutritional assessment, purchased the vitamins and minerals she needed, and instructed her on how, when and why she should take them. Next I prepared all her meals: nonfat, vegetarian fresh food breakfast, lunch and dinner. Foremost in the regimen however, was the Lymphatic Massage on a daily basis.

She spent two weeks with me. In her second week she walked seven blocks to the grocery store and back with two bags of groceries under her arms. When she arrived at the apartment, she sat for just a moment and then said, "Well, I guess I'll clean up the house!" I said, "Mom, do you realize what you have just done?" The look of surprise and amazement on her face at that moment made me know that I had embarked upon a journey that was at once awe inspiring and humbling. I was thankful that in some small measure I was able to return the love and comfort my mother had given me.

When she returned home to Cleveland, she saw her doctor and he exclaimed, "My God woman, what have you been doing? Your blood pressure is normal for the first time in four years." With only a mother's pride, she told him of her son, the nutritional massage doctor. He replied, "Well, whatever you have been doing, you should keep on doing it!"

I am thankful to my mom for putting me the right track and helping me stay on it. The Lymphatic Massage helped me to put my mother on the right track to health and wellness.

CASE #3: ELDERLY LADY ON TWO CANES

When I first met Ms. Jones, she was in the office of an obese gentleman who sold nutritional supplements for weight loss. I was dressed rather casually wearing my favorite green beret. When I saw her lack of coordination, I suggested that the Lymphatic Massage may be of benefit to her. She replied, "What is that?" I told her that in Europe, it is called Manual Lymph Drainage. She said, "I don't know Honey, I think I want to keep all my lymphs. I feel drained enough!" I smiled and assured her that she would not lose anything and it could help her. She said, "Well, I'm on my last legs and I'm willing to try anything to help me now."

The next day she arrived at my office walking on two canes. I helped her to fill out the intake forms, because she had difficulty with her eyesight. Then I helped her into the treatment room and onto the table. After the Lymphatic, I was writing my observations in her chart, when she came out of the treatment room. She looked over my shoulder and remarked, "I can read what you are writing from all the way over here!" Then she said, "You know, I think my balance is better too!"

I explained that the fluid in the ocular socket and inside the eyeball is lymphatic fluid. The pressure exerted by the fluid could change the shape of the eyeball and thereby affect her vision. I continued to elaborate on how the fluid in the inner ear was also lymphatic fluid and when in balance, it could affect a person's equilibrium. She then paid her fee and walked out of the office.

As I went into the treatment room to prepare for the next client, I saw her two canes propped up against the wall. I retrieved them and ran out to the parking lot to hand them to her through her car window. She never again came to the office with any kind of walking aid.

Her brother, who was amazed at her progress, paid for the remainder of her treatments. He said to her, "You had better let that man keep on rubbing on you if it does you this much good!" She became a regular client and continued to improve with each treatment of Lymphatic Massage.

CASE #4: YOUNG CHILD WITH ECZEMA

When his mother brought Alex to me, he was about two and a half years old. He was covered in gauze, wrapped up like a mummy. When we pealed off the layers of gauze wrappings, his skin was so covered with eczema that it would crack and bleed. I was impressed by his mother's trust in my and amazed by his courage. I started Lymphatic Massages three times per week. It took a lot of treatments. However, by the time we had reached 26, this little boy look like the model for the Ivory Snow baby with clear blue eyes, clear milky white skin, pink rosy cheeks, and a bright, cheerful disposition.

About a week after that, his father came to the office to talk to me. He said, "Dr. Brown, I don't understand what you are doing, but I can't argue with success! You are the only who has helped my child." He said, "thank you", and then shook my hand. Health never looked better than on that child, and success never felt better than that handshake! Once again I experienced the magnificent rewards of the Lymphatic Massage!

CASE #5: CORPORATE EXECUTIVE WITH CHRONIC FATIGUE

When John came to my office, he seemed very apprehensive, almost ashamed of his condition. He believed his executive status with his company was in jeopardy due to the chronic fatigue. His colleagues had accused him of malingering and he did not want anyone to know that he suffered from chronic fatigue syndrome. I suggested that he have a minimum of ten treatments with the first three within 24 to 48 hours apart and the remainder on a weekly basis. He agreed to this regimen.

By his seventh treatment, the change was remarkable. He stated that he had more energy than he had in the sixteen years he had suffered with this malady. By the time he had his tenth Lymphatic Massage, he felt he was new man. Then he asked the question, "What now? When do I have to come back?" I replied, "Well John, you will know when you need to return." He looked somewhat puzzled at first and then said, "OK!"

I saw John some two and one half years later. He called and said he had a cold and thought he ought to have a tune-up of three treatments in a row. He had been symptom free for two and one half years and it was clear that he had reached a better level of understanding of his internal balance gained through Lymphatic Massage.

We did the three treatments and all his cold and flu symptoms abated. He was off again to face his corporate challenges with vigor, vitality and confidence through Lymphatic Massage.

CASE #6: STUDENT WITH STREP THROAT

It is interesting to note how even those of us who are aware of the healing power of Lymphatic Massage sometimes forget. Case in point, my Tai-Chi instructor, a very insightful and spiritual individual and also a student of Lymphatic Massage. We happened to meet again after several years, and he could barely speak. He had been suffering with a sore throat for at least a week when we talked. He said, "I was thinking about taking some antibiotics, nothing else seems to work." I said, "Why don't I give you a Lymphatic?" He replied, "Thank you, I don't know why I hadn't thought of that myself."

Even after all these years, I am still awestruck by the power of the Lymphatic Massage. Within two treatments, all symptoms were completely gone! As we did Tai-Chi together the next morning, he said, "I am completely amazed at how fast I recovered after just two Lymphatics! Thanks Doc!" I silently thanked God for allowing me to participate in the miracle of Lymphatic Massage.

CASE #7: CALIFORNIA LADY WITH SEVERE P.M.S.

In 1982, I had just learned how to do the Lymphatic and other than my teacher, I had to find someone to practice on. When I met Mrs. G., I was very impressed with her equanimity, poise and grace. At the time, I had no idea that she suffered so severely. The week before her time, during her cycle and the week after, she spent in bed. I convinced her and another friend (a former real estate associate) to allow me to practice on them.

Dr. Childs had told me that this technique of Lymphatic Massage would help to balance hormones, but at this time I was merely refining my technique. To my surprise, Mrs. G. called me one day and said, "Bill, I am sitting here waiting to suffer, and it's not happening. I did not even know it was my time until I started to spot. Thank you so much!"

The next day I heard from Mrs. G's husband. He came into the office and asked for me. When I came out, he shook my hand and said, "I just want to thank you for giving my wife back to me!" I stood there once again humbled and awestruck at the power of the Lymphatic Massage.

CASE #8: THE PRIEST WITH MANIC DEPRESSION

Now when Father Smith came to me for a Lymphatic Massage, he often says to me, " I would like to have a Lymphatic because I feel sad or a little depressed." I, of course, would give him a treatment. Then I would attempt to explain why he feels so much better afterward from a clinical perspective, an explanation he requested as a professional in the field of psychiatric therapy.

"You see Father," I would say, "beyond the loving touch of this technique, it affects the neurohormones in the brain, particularly serotonin. When this neurohormone is not present in adequate amounts in the brain, depression sets in. When this hormone is elevated it changes your mood positively."

Father Smith had been treated with Librium for seven years and, with the help of Lymphatic Massage, was able to drastically reduce his dosage (under his medical doctor's supervision). Each and every treatment he received elevated his mood and lasted longer. He was finally able to move away from the drug regimen with the help of specific nutrient therapy and Lymphatic Massage.

I still have a picture of Father Smith in my mind, as he would leave my treatment room. His hair would be slightly disheveled and a slight smile on his face as he went out to share God's love and light with his parishioners.

CASE #9: RETIRED AKRON RUBBER TIRE FACTORY WORKER

When Mr. Sam first came to see me, the first thing I noticed was his ruddy complexion and his friendly smile. Beyond that, Mr. Sam had open sores in his scalp the size of quarters, and necrotic tissue covering his ankles that looked to be the color of black rubber. I started the Lymphatic treatments scheduling the first three in one week and then bi-weekly.

This condition took some time to mitigate, to say the least. I combined a specific nutritional program of whole foods, and vitamin and mineral therapy with the Lymphatic regimen. Within approximately sixteen treatments, the sores in his scalp had completely disappeared. The necrotic tissue around his ankles had also vanished! His skin had become as smooth and supple as a teenager.

I said to him, "Mr. Sam, have you noticed the condition of your skin lately?" He replied, "You bet I have Doc! You don't think I'm driving fifty miles one way for nothing?" We laughed out loud together. Once again I was joyously thankful to be a small part of God's healing with love and light through the Lymphatic Massage.

CASE #10: PREGNANT WOMAN FROM 1ST TRIMESTER THROUGH DELIVERY AND BREAST FEEDING

When Cathy first came to me, she had recently discovered her pregnancy. She was suffering severe morning sickness. After two treatments of the Lymphatic Massage, all symptoms of morning sickness were abated. We continued the treatments through the second and third trimester of her pregnancy. In the course of her pregnancy, the lower back pain and fluid retention in the legs, which so often accompanies the increase of weight, were also completely eliminated. Through the consistent application of Lymphatic Massage, the course of the pregnancy was far less traumatic. Furthermore, the delivery was much easier and there was no postpartum depression.

While breast feeding her healthy new baby, she developed mastitis (inflammation of the breast). Her breast became hardened and painful. Once again, Lymphatic Massage came to the rescue. After only two treatments, her breast returned to normal and she could resume breast feeding with no further complications. I was again thankful to be of service to God in support of the feminine creative principle and newborn humanity with the Lymphatic Massage.

CASE # 11: MAN WITH DIABETES

When John came into the office, I asked if he had diabetes. He responded yes. So we checked his blood sugar before the treatment and it was an astounding 296. Normal blood sugar ranges from 80 to 100. After the treatment we rechecked his blood sugar and it had dropped to 167. The amazing thing about the lymphatic Massage is that it stimulates the body to seek balance in all areas.

CASE # 12: MAN WITH DIABETES

Ray came into the office and I asked if he had diabetes. He responded yes. So we checked his blood sugar before the treatment and it was a mere 77. After the lymphatic treatment his blood sugar was 90. Both high blood sugar and low blood sugar are functions of the same root cause. Once again it was demonstrated that lymphatic Massage stimulates the body to balance on the organ level, on the emotional level and on the spiritual level.

"There is provision in nature for all the ills of man and a remedy for every disease."

Kloss

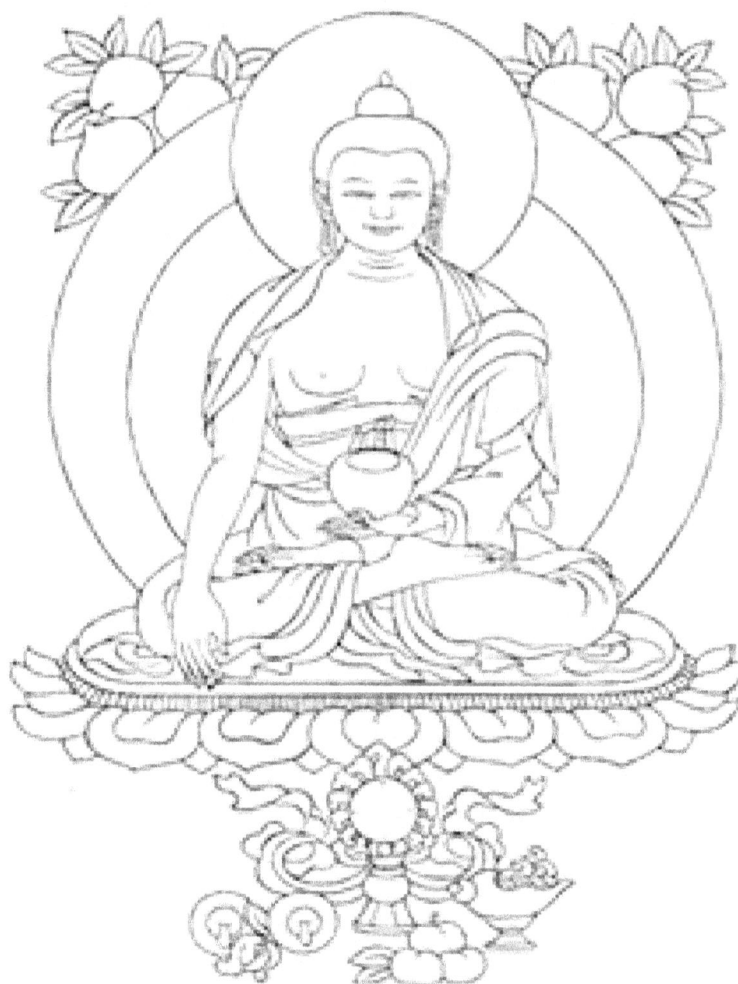

PART FOUR

INDEX OF BOOKS WRITTEN ON THERAPEUTIC MASSAGE
IN LYMPHATIC DISORDERS

1. Asdonk, J.; Bartetzko-Asdonk,C.
    (Diagnosis and general directions to physical therapy with post-mastectemic, chronic progressive arm lymphedema.) (In German with English summary) 1980. Zeitscrift fur Lymphologie. 4(2): 51-66.

    Addresses diagnosis and treatment of mild and severe uncomplicated lymphedema of the arm. Treatment methods include massage.

2. Asdonk, J.
    (Improvement of circulation by manual drainage of lymph.) (In French) 1978. Experientia [Supplement]. (33): 9-10.

3. Asdonk, J.
    (Lymphatic drainage by massage. Mechanism of action, indications, and contraindications.) (In German)
    1975 June 10. Zeitschrift fur Allgemeinmedizin. 51(16): 751-753.

    Argues that manual lymphatic drainage is a special massage method, which favors drainage via the blood vessels and lymphatics, but it is contraindicated in "malignant and highly virulent inflammatory conditions."

4. Asdonk, J.
    (Myogeloses, their pathogenesis and their lymph drainage, heat and exercise therapy).
    (In German with English summary)
    1985 June. Zeitschrift fur Lymphologie. 9(1): 30-37.

    Discusses the pathophysiology of myogeloses, which he states are nonspecific mesenchymal reactions with slight inflammatory symptoms which frequently arise due to capillary hypoxemia. Further discusses pathologic indications and recommends manual lymphatic drainage, in various states and combinations as the primary treatment.

5. Asdonk, J.
    (Physical lymph drainage and therapy of edema in chronic venous insufficiency.) (In German with English summary)
    1981 December. Zeitschrift fur Lymphologie. 5(2): 107-111.

6. Badger, C.
    The Swollen Limb.
    1986. Nursing Times. 82(31): 40-41.

    Discusses the current state of knowledge concerning the cause and control of lymphedema. Discusses an innovative British treatment program for patients with

The Touch That Heals

lymphedema due to cancer surgery or radiotherapy. Treatment no longer relies on diuretics, which reduce swelling at the price of causing dehydration. Instead, a variety of mechanical compression devises and/or massage are applied, as each case warrants.

7.   Bardychev, MS.
(Local radiation injuries and their combined treatment.) (In Russian)
1982. Meditsinskaia Radiologiia. 27(11): 44-49.

8.   Bargellesi, E.; Cappellaro, G.: Ricci, G.
(Lymphedema following mastectomy: treatment by compression and iontophoresis.) (In Italian with French and English summaries)
1984. Riabilitzaione. 17(3): 163-166.

9.   Bilancini, S.; Lucchi, M.
("Depletion" in the treatment of lymphedema of the lower extremeties.) (In French with English summary)
1987 April/June. Phlebologie. 40(2): 537-540.

      Discusses a two stage treatment program for lymphedema, which involves edema reduction and prevention of its recurrence. Stage two involves some contention, with various camps favoring manual lymphatic drainage, pressotherapy or wrapping and immersion in mercury. They advocate a method of their own based on clinical experience with 187 patients suffering from moderate edema of the lower extremities, but the abstract does not say what it consists of.

10.   Bolhmann, R.
(Treatment of lymphatic drainage.) (In French)
1971 October. Zeitschrift fur Krankenpflege. 64(10); 353.

      Offers nursing perspectives on massage as a treatment for lymphedema.

11.   Bollinger, A.
(New aspects of lymphedema.) (In German with English summary)
1985 June 15. Schweizerische Medizinische Wochenschrift. 115(24): 86-843.

      Reviews the current state of knowledge regarding the diagnosis and treatment of primary and secondary lymphedema. Discusses drug treatment and physiotherapy. Argues that combined physiotherapy with tight bandages and stockings, massage and the use of pneumatic devices for intermittent compression, considerably reduces the edema and renders surgery unnecessary in most patients.

12.   Borcsok, E.; Foldi, K.; Wittlinger, G.; Foldi, M.
(Treatment of acute experimental lymphostatic edema with vitamins, with vitamin-like natural substances, and with massage.) (In German)
1971. Angiologica. 8(1): 31-42.

13. Browse, NL.
     The diagnosis and management of primary lymphedema.
     1986 January. Journal of Vascular Surgery. 3(1); 181-184.

     Argues that although the clinical features of lymphedema are often distinctive, diagnosis ought to be confirmed by a diagnostic test. He proposes and explains his choice of such a test; isotopic lymphography. Discusses treatment alternatives. Claims the mainstay of edema reduction consists of regular elevation, massage and external compression with elastic stockings. Pneumatic massage devices are also helpful. Discusses surgical alternatives for complicated or refractory edema.

14. Brunner, U.; Wirth, W.
     (Dye test and lymphangiography in the evaluation of the etiolog and therapy of post-traumatic lymphedema in the legs.) (In German)
     1971 September 18. Schweizerische Medizinische Wochenschrfit 101(37): 1354-1358.

     Discusses the cause, diagnosis and treatment of lymphedema, including massage.

15. Calnan, J.S.; Pflug, J.J.; Reis, N.D.; Taylor, L.M.
     Lymphatic pressures and the flow of lymph.
     1970 October. British Journal of Plastic Surgery. 23(4): 305-317.

     Discusses the physiology of the lymphatic system and the effect of massage on the movement of lymphatic fluid.

16. (Cases from edema consultation.) (In German)
     1981 December. Zeitschrift fur Lymphologie 5(2): 83-89.

     Discusses various causes and clinical presentations of edema, including breast cancer, tongue cancer and varicose veins. Depicts various treatments including surgery, drugs and massage.

17. Casley-Smith, J.R.; Bjoerlin, M.O.
     Some parameters affecting the removal of oedema by massage, mechanical or manual.
     (Conference Paper)
     Paper presented at the Tenth International Congress of Lymphology, Adelaide, South Australia, August 26-September 2, 1985. 1985. Freiburg, West Germany: International Society for Lymphology.

18. Chekalina, S.I.; Guseva, L.I.
     (Blood coagulation disorders after radiotherapy and their treatment.) (InRussian)
     1981. Meditsinskaia Radiologiia. 26(4); 48-51.

     Studies the effect of radiotherapy on homoeostatic mechanisms in 55 patients being treated for various forms of cancer. All had radiation induced dysfunction blood and lymph circulation. Treatment consisted of exercise therapy, drugs and massage.

19. Cluzan, R.; Miserey, G.; Barrey, P.; Alliot, F.

(Principles and results of physiotherapeutic therapy in mechanical lymphatic insufficiency of secondary or primary origin.) (In French with English summary). 1988 April/June. Phlebologie. 41(2): 401-408.

> Discusses the physiotherapy of edemas of mechanical lymphatic insufficiency/lymphedema. Treatment consists of manual lymphatic drainage, volumetric reduction by wrapping with bandages and exercise, and maintenance of the result by wearing a retention device. Argues that primary lymphedema usually responds less favorably to treatment than does the secondary factor.

20. Davy, V.; Conolly, W.B.; Masman, A.
Clinical evaluation of the Masman pressure unit in the reduction of limb oedema.
1976. Australian Journal of Physiotheraphy. 22(4); 157-160.

> Discusses treatment of edema by mechanical massage device.

21. DeCuyper, H.; Hapers, F.
(Prevention and physical therapy of the oedematous arm after mastectomy and radiotherapy: a review article.) (In Dutch with English summary)
1978. Journal Belge De Medecine Physique et de Rehabilitation. 1(4); 288-310.

> Treatment alternatives addressed include iontophoresis and massage.

22. Dini, D.; Bianchini, J.; Massa, T.; Fassio, T.
(Treatment of upper limb lymphedema after mastectomy with escine and levo-thyrozine.) (In Italian with English summary)
1981 September 22. Minerva Medica. 72(35): 2319-2322.

> Discusses the results of 70 cases with post-mastectomy lymphedema in which two drugs were applied by massage in postural drainage, ionophoresis or pressotherapy, as the merits of each case decided.

23. Dupuis-Deltor.
(Physiotherapy of swollen arms. Treatment by massage and functional rehabilitation.) (In French)
1967 November. Journal de Radiologie D'Electrologie et de Medecine Nucleaire. 48(11): 808-809.

> Treatment alternatives discussed for secondary post-mastectomy lymphedema included massage and exercise therapy.

24. Dustmann, H.O.
(Diagnosis, differential diagnosis and therapy of lymphedema.) (In German with English summary)
1982 February. Zeitschrift fur Ortthopadie und Ihre Grenzgebiete. 120(1): 76-82.

Discusses the characteristics of various lymphedemas of the legs encountered in clinical practice, and pragmatics of diagnosis. Discusses various treatment alternatives. Surgery is recommended, but its inconsistent successfulness and incidence of complications is mentioned also. Claims that proper conservative treatment of massive lymphedemas consists of Van Der Molen's tube method, intermittent cuff pressure and manual lymphatic drainage. These methods are described in detail, as are disadvantages and risks of theses methods.

25.   Fischer, M.
(Thirty years of manual lymph drainage according to Vodder. A special form of massage for decompression of tissue.) (In German)
1967 February 20. Landazart. 43(5): 219-220.

>   Discusses the use of massage in the treatment of edema related to migraine and tooth diseases.

26.   Flowers, K.R.
String wrapping versus massage for reducing digital volume.
1988 January. Physical Therapy. 69(1): 57-59.

>   Conducted a clinical study to determine the relative effectiveness of two common methods of treating hand edema; retrograde massage and string wrapping. 56 digits on the hands of 14 subjects were studied.

27.   Foldi, M.
Anatomical and physiological basis for physical therapy of lymphedema.
1978. Experientia [Supplement]. (33): 15-18.

>   Discusses massage as the primary treatment.

28.   Foldi, M.
(Chronic lymphedema.) (In German)
1982 May 20. Foretschritte der Medizin. 100(19): 877-880.

>   Discusses the pathology and treatment of chronic lymphedema. Treatment consists of exercise therapy, massage and postural modificiation.

29.   Foldi, M.
(Lymphedema.) (In Dutch)
1979. Nederlands Tijdschrift voor Fysiotherapie. 89(2): 28-31.

>   Discusses treatment via massage and compression bandages.

30.   Foldi, M..
(Lymphedema of the arm after mastectomy.) (In German with English summary)
1980 May 8. Fortschritte der Medizin. 98(17); 672-678.

Argues that every lymphedema requires treatment. The first treatment to be tried ought to be a conservative complex "physical decongestion therapy", which may include massage, bandages and elevation. If this approach fails, surgery must be considered; these alternatives are discussed.

31.   Foldi, M.
(Lymphedema: how should lymphedema not be treated? Operative treatment of edema.) (In German)
1983. Gynakologische Rundschau. 23(3): 216-219.

Discusses surgical treatment and the use of diuretics, and their adverse effects. Addresses a conservative treatment which consists of massage and compression bandages.

32.   Foldi, M.
(Lymphedema of the limbs and genitals. V. Complex physical decongestion.) (In German)
1981. Monatskurse fur die Arztliche Fortbildung. 31(11): 436-442.

Discusses conservative treatment in the form of ultrasonics, compression dressings and massage.

33.   Foldi, M.
Lymphology today.
1983 February. Anigology. 34(2): 84-90.

Provides an overview of the physiology of the lymphatic system, and treatment alternatives, including surgery, exercise therapy, compression bandages, elevation and massage.

34.   Foldi, M.; Foldi, E.
(Therapy of lymphedema.) (In German)
1980 May 23. Medizinische Welt. 31(21): 801-806.

Discusses treatment alternatives which include surgery, compression bandages and massage.

35.   Foldi, M.
(Veno-lymphatic connections. Physiopathology. Clinical picture.) (In French with English summary)
1981 January/March. Phlebologie. 34(1): 111-115.

Investigates the mechanism by which the edema observed in chronic venous insufficiency develops. Describes in detail the pathophysiology and clinical presentations. With respect to therapy, recommends the advantages of gentle massage as a physical decongestant.

36.   Godart, S.; Leduc, A.;, Delacave, G.
(The influence of massage of the lymphatic vessels on the progression of lymph.) (In French)
1973. Angeiologie. 25(5): 214-218.

37.   Gorshkov, S.Z.; Podzharskaya, E.E.
(Conservative treatment of elephantiasis of the extremeties.) (In Russian)
1974. Sovetskaia. Meditsina. 37(12): 102-105.

      Discusses the alternatives for effectively treating this disorder. Advocates a complex conservative treatment, which is described in detail. Therapeutic measures include compression bandages, massage, physiotherapy, and diuretic and corticosteroid pharmaceutical agents.

38.   Gournay, J.
(Lymphostasis of the venous wall. Therapeutic implications.) (In French with English summary)

      Argues that lymphedema has to be treated in the same way that venous insufficiency of the lower extremities has to be treated by reduction. Surgery is mentioned as a last resort. Massage is mentioned as an aid to reduction.

39.   Grabois, M.

Rehabilitation of the postmastectomy patient with lymphedema.
1976 March/Aril. CA A Cancer Journal for Clinicians. 26(2): 75-79.

      Treatment alternatives addressed include compression bandages, massage, and, as a last resort, surgery.

40.   Gray, B.
Management of limb oedma in advanced cancer.
1987. Nursing Times. 83(49) 39-41.

      Discusses a treatment program implemented in Great Britain, but claimed to be of American origin, designed to treat lymphedema associated with advanced, terminal cancer, which can of itself adversely affect a patients quality of life. The 8 day program consists of use of an elastic containment garment and proximal massage, followed by pneumatic compression interspersed with fluid mobility exercises. The pragmatics of the program are discuss in detail.

41.   Gregl, A.
(Arm lymphography: technique; indication and results; side effects.) (In German)
1976. Folia Angiologica. 24 (½): 30-34.

      Discusses the use of wrist massage as apart of the technique for conducting a diagnostic test.

42. Gruffaz, J.
(Manual lymphatic drainage.) (In French with English summary)
1985. Journal des Maladies Vascularies. 10(Supplement A): 1870191.

> Argues that manual lymphatic drainage, a non-invasive for the treatment of lymphedema, has yet to compellingly demonstrate its effectiveness against other techniques. Two factors further inhibit its usefulness: there are very few such therapists available and that French national social security does not recognize the method for financial reimbursement.

43. Heytmanek, G.; Kubista, E.
(Therapy of postoperative lymphedema in breast cancer: lymph drainage.)
(In German with English summary)
1988 June. Geburtshilfe und Frauenheilkundle. 48(6): 433-435.

> Argued that as lymphedema is a complication affecting approximately 10% of surgical interventions with modified radical mastectomy, a prophylactic aid must be developed to address this problem. Claim their clinical department tested and obtained good results using both manual lymphatic drainage and mechanical massage devices for expressing lymph.

44. Hoffmann, A.; Petzoldt, D.
(Manual lymph drainage.) (In German with English summary)
1978 September. Hautarzt. 29(9): 463-466.

> Argues that manual lymphatic drainage is a specialized method of massage, often used for "cosmetical purposes" to treat lymphedema associated with rheumatism and trigeminal neuralgia. Thoroughly describes the method, its mode of action, clinical indications, and results to be expected.

45. Horn, H.G.
(Manual lymph drainage as part of a health gymnastic exercise program.) (In German)
1984. Krankengymnastik. 36(7): 458-459.

> Presents a case report on the efficacy of manual lymphatic drainage in a treatment program.

46. Hornbacher, W.
(Thrombophebitis and arthritis as well as several other indications for lymph drainage treatment.) (In German)
1974. April 20. Zeitschrift fur Allgemeinmedizin. 50(11): 530-531.

> Discusses the application of manual lymphatic drainage to the treatment of arthritis and thrombophlebitis.

47. Hutzschenreuter, P.; Brummer, H.
(Lymphangiomotricity and tissue pressure.) (In German with English summary)

1986 December. Zeitschrift fur Lymphologie. 10(2): 55-57.

48.   Hutzschenreuter, P.; Brummer, H.
       Pressure effects in subcutaneously given hematoma under condition of locally applied ice bags or of compression bandage or massage for lymphatic drainage according to Vodder. (Meeting Abstract)
       1987. International Journal of Sports Medicine. 8(2): 161.

49.   Imamaliev, A.S.; Lirtsman, V.M.; Nikitin, S.E.; Shkrabov, B.S.; Kisin, B.M.
       (Use of pneumo-massage for treating post-traumatic edema of the lower extremities.) (In Russian)
       1983 February. Ortopediia Travmatologiia I Protezirovanie. (2): 55-56.

50.   Ito, T.; Ichimura, H.; Nishizawa, K.
       (Apparatus for undulatory air massage used in treatment of edematous swelling of the arm after radical mastectomy.) (In Japanese with German summary)
       1977. Hirosaki Medical Journal. 29(1): 132-142.

       Discusses beneficial results obtained following treatment of 11 patients with arm edema following radical mastectomy.

51.   Ito, T.; Ichimura, H.: Nichizawa, K.; Fukushi, M.; Hatakeyama, T.; Hanada, N.; Shinozaki, T.; Kure, T.; Ishizuka, E.
       (The experience of the use of the wave-form air massage apparatus for edema of the arms following radical mastectomy.) (In Japanese)
       1977. Hirosake Igaku. 29(1): 134-142.

       Discusses the results of a clinical study of 11 patients with post-mastectomy lymphedema of the arm. Claims 8 of 11 patients shows reduction of edema and improvement of subjective complaints following treatment with a device for wave-form air massage. Argues that cases in which a complex treatment was applied, consisting of wave-form air massage, manual massage, elevation of the arms, and use of elastic stockings fared better than those which received only wave-form air massage. Case in which manual massage and "Hari-therapy" were applied together showed a prominent and long lasting effect.

52.   Kuhnke, E.
       (Autonomic changes in lymph drainage.) (In German)
       1987 December. Zeitschrift fur Lymphologie. 11(2): 59-62.

       Discusses the pathophysiology of lymphedema and its relationship to autonomic nervous system pathology. Addresses the innervation of smooth muscle and its problems. Proposes drainage via massage.

53.   Kuhnke, E.

(Evidence for efficacy of therapeutic lymph drainage: demonstration in arm edema following breast amputation.) (In German with French and English summaries)
1979. Phlebologie und Proktologie. 8(2): 139-152.

Claims to present results of a statistically significant beneficial effect due to manual lymphatic drainage in the case of 29 outpatients treated at the clinic of one such practitioner.

54.   Kuhnke, E.
(Statistical demonstration of the Vodder-Asdonk method of manual drainage of lymph.)
(In German)
1978. Experientia [Supplement]. (33): 33-46.

Discusses the physiology of the lymphatic system, and causes of lymphedema. Addresses treatment via this method for secondary post-mastectomy lymphedema.

55.   Kurtz, W.; Wittlinger, G.; Litmanovitch, Y.I.; Romanoff, H.; Pfeifer, Y.: Tal, E.; Sulman, F.G.
Effect of manual lymph drainage massage on urinary excretion of neurohormones and minerals in chronic lymphedema.
1978 October. Angiology. 29(10): 762-764.

A clinical study of 29 patients with chronic lymphedema of diverse original mostly affecting the lower extremities who were treated with manual lymphatic drainage indicated significant changes in urinary neurohormone excretion, which did not prove the case with respect to secretion of 17-KS, thyroxine, various minerals and creatinine. The authors argue that these findings underscore the importance of epinepherine and norepinepherine release by manual lymphatic drainage, which improves circulation. But they claim that as their findings indicate the involvement of histamine and perhaps serotonin in lymphedema formation, combines MLD massage with antihistamine and antiserotonin treatment might prove more effective

56.   Kurz, W.; Kurz, R.; Litmanovitch, Y.I.; Romanoff, H.; Pfeifer, Y.; Sulman, F.G.
Effect of manual lymph drainage massage on blood components and urinary neurohormones in chronic lymphedema.
1981 Feburary. Angiology. 32(2): 119-127.

57.   Leduc, O.; Bourgois, P.; Leduc, A.
(Experimental evaluation of the influence of manual lymphatic drainage using isotopic lymphography.) (In French)
1988. Annales de Kinisiterapie. 15(4): 153-158.

58.   Leduc, A.; Lemense, L.
(Manual drainage of lymph in cellulitis of venous origin.) (In French)
1978. Experientia [Supplement]. (33): 47-50.

59.   Leitner, G.

(Results of treatment with mechanical expressors and studies of their efficacy.) (In German)
1981 December. Zeitschrift fur Lymphologie. 5(2): 118-122.

Discusses use of massage instrumentation in the treatment of lymphedema.

60.   Lewis, J.M.; Wald, E.R.
Lymphedema praecox.
1984 May. Journal of Pediatarics. 104(5): 641-648.

Provides a review of the literature and case reports on the pathophysiology and treatment of pediatric and adolescent lymphedema and lymphangitis. Treatment consists of diuretics and massage.

61.   Lindemayr, H.; Santler, R.; Jurecka, W.
(Compression therapy of lymphedema.) (In German with English summary)
1980 May 30. Munchener Medizinische Wochenschrift. 122(22): 825-828.

Argues that although microsurgical techniques have grown very sophisticated and enable functioning lympho-venous anastomoses to be formed, such interventions are usually inappropriate when the extremity has already been irreparably damaged by edema. In such cases, compression therapy is still the treatment of choice. Its mode of action and clinical indications are discussed. Argues that manual lymphatic drainage provides acceptable results only in the early, still reversible stages of the condition.

62.   Manuel Nogueras, F.
(Prophylazis and treatment of upper limb edema after radical mastectomy.) (In Spanish)
1975. Cirugia Espanola. 29(2): 177-195.

63.   Masman, A.R.; Conolly, W.B.
Intermittent pressure in the management of post-traumatic oedema and lymphedema. The rationale and description of a new method.
1976. Medical Journal of Australia. 1(4): 87-89.

Discusses the rationale for use and effectiveness, in a clinical study of 63 patients with lymphedema, of an intermittent pressure devise claimed to be effective in reducing limb girt, and at low cost.

64.   Mayer, M.; Colon, J.; Blondet, R.
(Chronic lymphedema after treatment for cancer of the breast without recurrence. Results after lymphatic drainage as used by Thompson.) (In French)
1973. Lyon Chirurgical. 69(6): 401-407.

Discusses a surgical drainage technique that was carried out in 6 patients. It was said that the procedure created an efferent lymphatic path with can be improved by muscle contraction and massage. Claims that reduction of edema continued from the second through the sixth month post-surgery, without complications.

65. Megret, G.
(Therapeutic principles of lymphostatis of the extremities.) (In French with English summary)
1982 April/June. Phlebologie. 35(2): 561-567.

Discusses classifications of lymphedema of the limbs, and describes channels of lymphatic return and their anatomical structure. Addresses in detail various treatment options and their implications: Medications, surgical techniques of increasing sophistication, and conservative methods, which seek to recover a physiological site for lymphatic reflux. Among the methods discussed are manual lymphatic drainage and compression.

66. Muller, R.
(Lymphostatic conditions of the lower extremities and their treatment.) (In German)
1963 August 16. Fortschritte der Medizin. 91(22): 891-896.

Discusses the diagnostic use of dyes, and treatment methods, including compression bandages, exercise therapy, diuretics, vitamins and massage.

67. Ohkuma, M.; Kishimoto, T.; Nakano, T.; Hirai, R.; Yamazaki, H.; Tezuka, T.
(Elephantiasis nostras.) (In Japanese)
1979. Runsho Hifuka. 33(8): 737-740.

Discusses the case of a 75 year old woman with this condition as a complication of radiation therapy. Discusses the clinical presentation and course of the condition to date. The patient was treated with massage, which yielded an ablation of her subjective symptoms.

68. Ohkuma, M.; Kurimoto, K.; Takahashi, Y.; Tezuka, T.
(Nonfamilial congenital lymphedema.) (In Japanese)
1981. Nishinihon Journal of Dematology. 43(5): 794-796.

Discusses the pathophysiolog and treatment of a six year old boy with congenital edema of the right cheek, genitalia and right lower limb. Treatment, which was ineffective, included compression, massage, elastic stockings and drugs.

69. Partsch, H.; Mostbeck, A.; Leitner, G.
(Experimental investigations of the effect of pressure-wave massage [Lymphapress] in lymphedema.) (In German with English summary)
1981 July. Zeitscrift fur Lymphologie. 5(1): 35-39.

An investigation of the effects of a massage by the Lymphapress device yielded a demonstrable reduction in limb girth and a decrease in albumin content of the tissues. However, there is an increase in local albumin content in lymphedema by overproportional water reduction. Thus, compression bandages should be applied between Lymphapress massages to maintain the effect.

70.   Partsch, H.; Mostbeck, A.; Leitner, G.
        (Experimental study of the effect of pressure-wave massage [Lymphapress] on lymphedema.) (In German with French and English summaries)
        1980. Phlebologie und Proktologie. 9(2): 124-128.

        This is essentially a repeat of what was done in number 69 and with the same findings.

71.   Pflug, J.
        (Physiopathology and treatment of lymphedema.) (In French)
        1974 October/December. Phlebologie. 27(4): 393-396.

        Treatment alternatives discussed include diuretics, surgery and massage.

72.   Richmand, D.M.; O'Donnell, T.F., Jr.; Zelikovski, A.
        Sequential pneumatic compression for lymphedema. A controlled trial.
        1985. Archives of Surgery. 120(10): 1116-1119.

        25 patients, 7 with upper extremity lymphedema and 18 with lower extremity lymphedema underwent 24 hours of treatment with a pneumatic compression device, which utilizes a short duration high pressure cycle that provides a sequential milking pattern to the limb through multiple compartments. All extremities showed a significant decrease in girth without elevation in serum muscle enzymes. The authors claim that the device rapidly and safely reduces edematous limbs.

73.   Ryan, T.J.; Mortimer, P.S.; Jones, R.L.
        Lymphatics of the skin. Neglected but important.
        1986 September. International Journal of Dermatology. 25(7): 411-419.

        This review articles discusses the anatomy and histology of these lymphatics, the pathophysiology of lymphatic disorders, and treatment alternatives, including compression bandages, exercise therapy, and massage.

74.   Schulthess, K.
        (Manual lymph drainage.) (In German)
        1971 November. Zeitschrift fur Krankenpflege. 64(11): 383.

        Offers nursing perspectives on use of this method in treatment.

75.   Selosse, E.
        (Vodder's manual lymph drainage in post-traumatic edema.) (In French)
        1981. Cahiers de Kinisitherapie. (90): 97-102.

76.   Serniuk, I.U.M.

(Edema and reduced mobility of the arm in complex rehabilitation of breast cancer patients.) (In Russian)
1981. Klinicheskaia Khirugiia. (5): 62-64.

Addresses the cases of 193 patients who underwent radical mastectomy. 115 developed edema of the arm. Early edema, occurring within five to six months after surgery, was recorded after surgery alone. Late edema, that occurring longer than six months after surgery, was predominant in patients who underwent both surgery and radiation therapy. Physical therapy, prednisone administration, and massage of the arm, the authors argued, provided effective rehabilitation of the patients with reduced mobility of the arm.

77.   Stillwell, G.K.
Management of arm edema. In Stoll, B.A. (Editor). **Breast cancer management; early and late.**
1977. Chicago. William Heinemann Medical Books.

Discusses the mechanisms of post-mastectomy edema, and modalities of treatment applied at the May Clinic in Rochester, MN. Treatment consisting of removal of fluid from the limb via elevation, massage and exercise; and impedance of fluid accumulation via external elastic support, are compared with other published methods.

78.   Stillwell, G.K.
Treatment of post-mastectomy lymphedema in humans: elevation, massage, exercise, elastic, elastic support, diuretics, antibiotics.
1969. Modern Treatment. 6(2): 396-412.

79.   Strauli, P.
The barrier function of lymph nodes. A review of experimental studies and their implications for cancer surgery.
1970. Aktuelle Probleme in der Chirurgie. 14: 161-176.

80.   Swedborg, I.
Effectiveness of combines methods of physiotherapy for post-mastectomy lymphedema.
1980. Scandinavian Journal of Rehabilitation Medicine. 12(2): 77-85.

Discussed a post-mastectomy physiotherapy program applied to 39 patients over six months to reduce the development of arm edema. Treatment techniques included massage, isometric exercises and an elastic sleeve. During the first week of daily treatment an 11-13% reduction in edema volume was observed, but during the subsequent three weeks the benefit was sharply reduced. To maintain volume reduction in the swollen arm, an elastic sleeve was applied, and during the four weeks that the sleeve was worn there was no significant increase in volume.

81.   Ter Horst, W.
(Manual lymph drainage and its criteria.) (In Dutch)
1978. Nederlands Tijdschrift voor Fysiotherapie. 89(2): 32-35.

82.   Ter Horst, W.
        (Manual lymph drainage: a form of therapy?) (In Dutch)
        1978. Nederlands Tijdschrift voor Fysiotherapie. 88(10): 252-253.

83.   Ti-Sheng, Z.; Wen-Yi, H.; Liang-Yu, H.; Wu-Yi, L.
        Heat and bandage treatment for chronic lymphedema of the extremities. Report of 1,045 cases.
        1984. Chinese Medical Journal. 97(8): 567-577.

        Also discusses the use of massage.

84.   Traissac, B.; Sagardoy, G.; Lucas, J.F.
        (Manual lymphatic drainage in angiology.) (In French with English summary)
        1988 April/June. Phlebologie. 41(2): 471-476.

        Argues that manual lymphatic drainage is an "easy therapeutic method but it requires a high level of technical ability" to be successfully applied. States that the method gives good results in congenital and acquired lymphedema, venous insufficiency, and some general diseases, such as headache and colitis.

85.   Truche, H.; Boutroux, Y.C.; Bouchet, J.Y.
        (Rehabilitation in venous and lymphatic peripheral diseases: principles and methods.)
        (In French with English summary)
        1985. Annales de Readaption et de Medecine Physique. 27(3/4): 337-345.

        States that the rehabilitation of lymphatic and venous diseases is based on the use of a combination of methods, including manual lymphatic drainage, active and passive muscular exercises, breathing reeducation, bath and mineral water therapy, elastic stockings, and practicing sports. Lymphedema is treated by manual lymphatic drainage, mechanical pressotherapy and high pressure elastic stockings.

86.   Valtonen, E.J.
        Treatment of lymphedema of the extremities following surgery and radiotherapy.)
        1967. Annales Chirugiae et Gynaecologiae Fenniae. 56(2): 144-148.

        Discusses treatments of post-operative complications of breast, genital and skin cancer with surgery, exercise therapy and massage.

87.   Vansudevan, S.V.; Melvin, J.L.
        Upper extremity edema control: rationale of the techniques.
        1979 August. American Journal of Occupational Therapy. 33(8): 520-523.

        Discusses the pathophysiology and treatment of upper extremity lymphedema. A conservative treatment program consists of elevation, massage, use of external compression devices and exercise. The author discusses physiologic rationale for the effectiveness of these methods.

88. Von Arnim, D.
(What is meant by "manual lymph drainage" according to Vodder?) (In German)
1970 April 24. Munchener MedizinischeWochenschrift. 112(17): 813-814.

89. Walby, R.
(Treatment of lymphedema with pulsator. How to help patients with lymphedema following breast cancer operations.) (In Norwegian with English summary)
1983 August 30. Tidsskrift for den Norske Legeforening. 103(24): 1697-1698.

  Treatment method addressed was mechanical vibration massage.

90. Yamazaki, Z.; Fujimori, Y.; Wada, T.; Togawa, T.; Yamakoshi, K.; Shimazu, H.
Admittance plethysmographic evaluation of undatory massage for the edematous limb.
1979. Lymphology. 12(1): 40-42.

91. Yamazaki, Z.; Idezuki, Y.; Nemoto, T.; Togawa, T.
Clinical experience over the last ten years using pneumatic massage therapy for edematous limbs.
1988 February. Angiology. 39(2): 154-163.

  Discusses the details of the treatment of more than 650 patients suffering from edematous limbs at a clinic, using a pneumatic massage device designed to displace stagnant lymph and venous blood toward the heart. The authors indicate generally satisfactory results, with significant reduction in limb girth, but only if other "conservative treatments" are applied in the intervals between pneumatic treatments.

92. Zanolla, R.; Monzeglio, C.; Balzarini, A.; Martino, G.
Evaluation of the results of three different methods of post-mastectomy lymphedema treatments.
1984 July. Journal of Surgical Oncology. 26(3): 210-213.

  60 past-mastectomy patients with secondary early edema were randomly assigned into three groups to determine the relative effectiveness of three methods of post-mastectomy lymphedema treatment: pneumatic massage with uniform pressure, pneumatic massage with varying pressure and manual lymphatic drainage. Results indicated a permanent statistically significant edema reduction with uniform pressure, pneumatic massage with varying pressure and manual lymphatic drainage, but not with differentiated pressure pneumatic massage.

Additional References Added for 2008 Edition:

1. Warwick, Roger; Peter L. Williams [1858] (1973). "Angiology (Chapter 6)", Gray's anatomy, illustrated by Richard E. M. Moore, Thirty-fifth Edition, London: Longman, 588—785.

2. Sloop, Charles H.; Ladislav Dory, Paul S. Roheim (March 1987). "Interstitial fluid lipoproteins". Journal of Lipid Research 28 (3): 225—237. PMID 3553402. Retrieved on 2008-07-07.

3.   Pepper, Michael S.; Michaela Skobe (2003-10-27). "Lymphatic endothelium :
      morphological, molecular and functional properties". The Journal of Cell Biology 163 (2):
      209-213. doi:10.1083/jcb.200308082. Retrieved on 2008-07-06.

4.   Shayan, Ramin; Achen, Marc G.; Stacker, Steven A. (2006). "Lymphatic vessels in cancer
      metastasis: bridging the gaps" 27 (9): 1729. doi:10.1093/carcin/bgl031. PMID 16597644.

5.   Baluk, Peter; Jonas Fuxe, Hiroya Hashizume, Talia Romano, Erin Lashnits, Stefan Butz,
      Dietmar Vestweber, Monica Corad, Cinzia Molendini, Elisabetta Dejana, and Donald M.
      McDonald (2007-09-10). "Functionally specialized junctions between endothelial cells of
      lymphatic vessels". Journal of Experimental Medicine 204 (10): 2349-2362. PMID 17846148.
      10.1084/jem.20062596. Retrieved on 2008-07-07.

6.   Rosse, Cornelius; Penelope Gaddum-Rosse [1962] (1997). "The Cardiovascular System
      (Chapter 8)", Hollinshead's Textbook of Anatomy, Fifth Edition, Philadelphia:
      Lippincott-Raven, 72—73. ISBN 0-397-51256-2.

7.   Venugopal, A.M.; Stewart, R.H.; Laine, G.A. & Quick, C.M. (2004), "Optimal Lymphatic
      Vessel Structure", 26th Annual International Conference of the IEEE, vol. 2, Engineering in
      Medicine and Biology Society, pp. 3700—3703.

8.   Goldsby, Richard; Kindt, TJ; Osborne, BA; Janis Kuby [1992] (2003). "Cells and Organs of
      the Immune System (Chapter 2)", Immunology, Fifth Edition, New York: W. H. Freeman and
      Company, 24—56. ISBN 07167-4947-5.

9.   Lymphedema, <http://www.merck.com/mmhe/sec03/ch037/ch037b.html>

10.   Ambrose, C. (2006). "Immunology's first priority dispute—An account of the 17th-century
      Rudbeck–Bartholin feud". Cellular Immunology 242: 1. doi:10.1016/j.cellimm.2006.09.004.

11.   Fanous, Medhat YZ; Anthony J Phillips, John A Windsor (2007). "Mesenteric Lymph: The
      Bridge to Future Management of Critical Illness". Journal of the Pancreas 8 (4): 374—399.
      Department of Internal Medicine and Gastroenterology ALMA MATER STUDIORUM -
      UNIVERSITY OF BOLOGNA. Retrieved on 2008-07-11.

12.   Flourens, P. (1859). "ASELLI, PECQUET, RUDBECK, BARTHOLIN (Chapter 3)", A
      History of the Discovery of the Circulation of the Blood. Rickey, Mallory & company,
      67—99. Retrieved on 2008-07-11.

13.   Eriksson, G. (2004). "Olaus Rudbeck as scientist and professor of medicine (Original article in
      Swedish)". Svensk Medicinhistorisk Tidskrift 8 (1): 39—44. Retrieved on 2008-07-11.

14.   "Disputatio anatomica, de circulatione sanguinis". Account of Rudbeck's work on lymphatic
      system and dispute with Bartholin. The International League of Antiquarian Booksellers.
      Retrieved on 2008-07-11.

Journal Articles

Jeltsch M., Kaipainen A., Joukov V., Meng X., Lakso M., Rauvala H., Swartz M., Fukumura D., Jain R.K., Alitalo K., Hyperplasia of lymphatic vessels in VEGF-C transgenic mice. Science. 1997; 276: 1423-5

Book chapters Ferrara N., Gerber H., The Vascular Endothelial Growth Factor Family. In: Ware J.A., Simons M. eds. Angiogenesis and Cardiovascular Disease. New York: Oxford University Press; 1999: 101-27.

Articles and Abstracts on Lymphatic Massage

1. Cooperative and redundant roles of VEGFR-2 and VEGFR-3 signaling in adult lymphangiogenesis., PubMed ID: 17210781, Date: April 2007

2. A driving force for change: interstitial flow as a morphoregulator. PubMed ID: 17141502 Date: January 2007

3. The incidence of symptomatic lower-extremity lymphedema following treatment of uterine corpus malignancies: a 12-year experience at Memorial Sloan-Kettering Cancer Center. PubMed ID: 16740298 Date: November 2006

4. Quantification of cerebrospinal fluid transport across the cribriform plate into lymphatics in rats. PubMed ID: 16793937 Date: November 2006

5. Contractile activity of lymphatic vessels is altered in the TNBS model of guinea pig ileitis. PubMed ID: 16675748 Date: October 2006

6. Vascular endothelial growth factor-A mediates ultraviolet B-induced impairment of lymphatic vessel function. PubMed ID: 17003502 Date: October 2006

7. Production of two novel monoclonal antibodies that distinguish mouse lymphatic and blood vascular endothelial cells. PubMed ID: 16685512 Date: October 2006

8. Contraction-initiated NO-dependent lymphatic relaxation: a self-regulatory mechanism in rat thoracic duct. PubMed ID: 16809357 Date: September 2006

9. Transfection of human hepatocyte growth factor gene ameliorates secondary lymphedema via promotion of lymphangiogenesis. PubMed ID: 16952986 Date: September 2006

10. Differentiation of lymphatic endothelial cells from embryonic stem cells on OP9 stromal cells. PubMed ID: 16690875 Date: September 2006

11. Indirect magnetic resonance lymphangiography in patients with lymphedema preliminary results in humans. PubMed ID: 16621396 Date: September 2006

12. Expression of the TAL1/SCL transcription factor in physiological and pathological vascular processes. PubMed ID: 16841371 Date: September 2006

13. Vascular endothelial growth factor-C accelerates diabetic wound healing. PubMed ID: 16936280 Date: September 2006

14. Lymphatic vessels in cancer metastasis: bridging the gaps. PubMed ID: 16597644 Date: September 2006

15. Transcapillary fluid balance consequences of missing initial lymphatics studied in a mouse model of primary lymphoedema. PubMed ID: 16675495 Date: July 2006

16. Transcapillary fluid balance consequences of missing initial lymphatics studied in a mouse model of primary lymphoedema. PubMed ID: 16675495 Date: July 2006

17. On the transendothelial passage of tumor cell from extravasal matrix into the lumen of absorbing lymphatic vessel. PubMed ID: 16730031 Date: July 2006

18. Functional interaction of VEGF-C and VEGF-D with neuropilin receptors. PubMed ID: 16816121 Date: July 2006

19. Predictive factors of response to intensive decongestive physiotherapy in upper limb lymphedema after breast cancer treatment: a cohort study. PubMed ID: 16752081 Date: July 2006

20. Distribution of lymphatic vessels in mouse thymus: immunofluorescence analysis. PubMed ID: 16541287 Date: July 2006

21. Generation and characterization of a mouse lymphatic endothelial cell line. PubMed ID: 16534603 Date: July 2006

22. Autologous morphogen gradients by subtle interstitial flow and matrix interactions. PubMed ID: 16603487 Date: July 2006

23. Inflammatory manifestations of experimental lymphatic insufficiency. PubMed ID: 16834456 Date: July 2006

24. VEGF and PlGF promote adult vasculogenesis by enhancing EPC recruitment and vessel formation at the site of tumor neovascularization. PubMed ID: 16754748 Date: July 2006

25. VEGF and PlGF promote adult vasculogenesis by enhancing EPC recruitment and vessel formation at the site of tumor neovascularization. PubMed ID: 16754748 Date: July 2006

26. Tumor-induced lymphangiogenesis: a target for cancer therapy? PubMed ID: 16497404 Date: June 2006

27. Randomized controlled trial of weight training and lymphedema in breast cancer survivors. PubMed ID: 16702582 Date: June 2006

28.   The forkhead transcription factors, Foxc1 and Foxc2, are required for arterial specification and lymphatic sprouting during vascular development. PubMed ID: 16678147 Date: June 2006

29.   Diagnosis and management of primary chylous ascites. PubMed ID: 16765248 Date: June 2006

30.   Endothelial cell biology: an update. 5th International Symposium on the Biology of Endothelial Cells. PubMed ID: 16732383 Date: June 2006

31.   Lymphatic vessel density as a prognostic indicator for patients with stage I cervical carcinoma. PubMed ID: 16733213 Date: June 2006

32.   Inhibition of active lymph pump by simulated microgravity in rats. PubMed ID: 16399874 Date: June 2006

33.   Structure function relationships in the lymphatic system and implications for cancer biology. PubMed ID: 16770531 Date: June 2006

34.   Lymphangiogenesis and expression of specific molecules as lymphatic endothelial cell markers. PubMed ID: 16800291 Date: June 2006

35.   Lymphatic zip codes in premalignant lesions and tumors. PubMed ID: 16740707 Date: June 2006

36.   Lymph node metastasis in breast cancer xenografts is associated with increased regions of extravascular drain, lymphatic vessel area, and invasive phenotype. PubMed ID: 16707438 Date: May 2006

37.   Imaging of lymphatic vessels in breast cancer-related lymphedema: intradermal versus subcutaneous injection of 99mTc-immunoglobulin. PubMed ID: 16632730 Date: May 2006

38.   Time course of angiogenesis and lymphangiogenesis after brief corneal inflammation. PubMed ID: 16670483 Date: May 2006

39.   Hepatocyte growth factor is a lymphangiogenic factor with an indirect mechanism of action. PubMed ID: 16424394 Date: May 2006

40.   Vascular endothelial growth factor (VEGF)/VEGF-C mosaic molecules reveal specificity determinants and feature novel receptor binding patterns. PubMed ID: 16505489 Date: April 2006

41.   Vascular endothelial growth factor (VEGF)/VEGF-C mosaic molecules reveal specificity determinants and feature novel receptor binding patterns. PubMed ID: 16505489 Date: April 2006

42.   A polysaccharide isolated from the medicinal herb Bletilla striata induces endothelial cells proliferation and vascular endothelial growth factor expression in vitro. PubMed ID: 16614890 Date: April 2006

43.   Lymphangiogenesis in the bone-implant interface of orthopedic implants: importance and consequence. PubMed ID: 16392126 Date: April 2006

44.   Onset of abnormal blood and lymphatic vessel function and interstitial hypertension in early stages of carcinogenesis. PubMed ID: 16585153 Date: April 2006

45.   Lymphatic or hematogenous dissemination: how does a metastatic tumor cell decide? PubMed ID: 16627996 Date: April 2006

46.   Signal transduction by VEGF receptors in regulation of angiogenesis and lymphangiogenesis. PubMed ID: 16336962 Date: March 2006

47.   Lymphscintigraphic evaluation of manual lymphatic drainage for lower extremity lymphedema. PubMed ID: 16724509 Date: March 2006

48.   Pulmonary air embolization inhibits lung lymph flow by increasing lymphatic outflow pressure. PubMed ID: 16569202 Date: March 2006

49.   Expression of lymphatic vascular endothelial hyaluronan receptor-1 (LYVE-1) in the human placenta. PubMed ID: 16569201 Date: March 2006

50.   Intratissular lymphaticovenous anastomoses demonstrated by perioperative intramuscular injection of 99mTC-colloids. PubMed ID: 16569204 Date: March 2006

"Men who are in earnest are not afraid of consequences."

Marcus Garvey

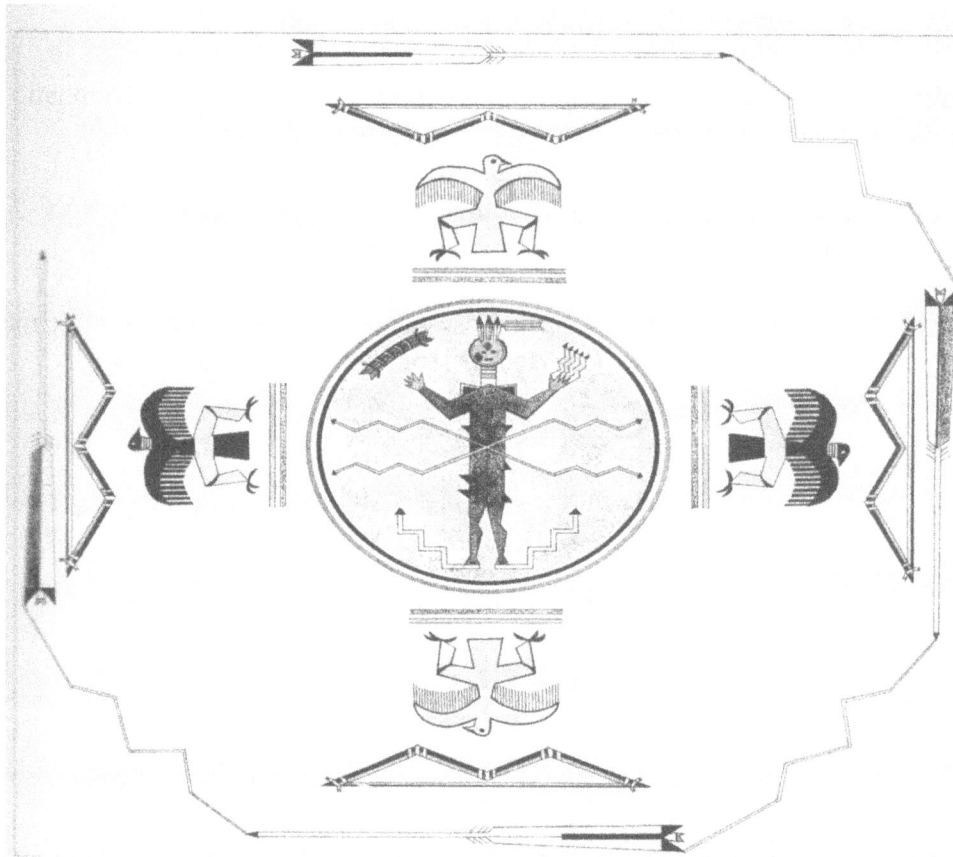

© Jose´ and Miriam Argüelles and
Shambala Publications, Inc. , 1972

PART FIVE

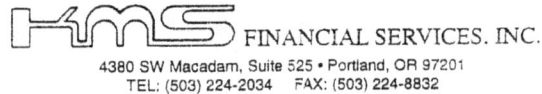

KMS FINANCIAL SERVICES. INC.

4380 SW Macadam, Suite 525 • Portland, OR 97201
TEL: (503) 224-2034   FAX: (503) 224-8832

June 24, 1998

Mr. Bill Brown
315 Willow Way
Sedona   AZ   86336

Dear Mr. Brown:

When I was at the Enchantment Resort, I took advantage of the spa by having a lymphatic massage administered by Mary Meyer. The results were so positive that after returning to Portland, I wrote to Mary asking her about the technique and where I might learn more about it.

She has indicated that you were her instructor and gave me your address.

Have you written about your technique or did you learn it from someone else who may have written a text on it?

I have had breast cancer and my right underarm lymph nodes were removed. As a Kaiser Permanente member I have availed myself of their treatments for lymphadema which is a combination of massage and exercise. But, I found Mary's treatment to be more long lasting. It would be great if I could refer my physical therapist to an additional methodology to the one Kaiser uses which was developed and has been used in Germany for many years, at least, so I understand.

If you have any references for me, I would appreciate receiving them.

Sincerely,

Nancy

Nancy Rangila, CFA, CFP
Financial Consultant

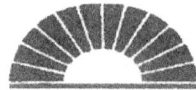

CASE WESTERN RESERVE UNIVERSITY

3/5/03

To Whom it may concern,

Dr. William Brown has given lectures in an elective forum to medical students at Case Western Reserve University School of Medicine. He is very knowledgeable in his field. His lectures on Lymphatic Drainage and Neurologic Integration were dynamic and well received by the students. His demonstrations were able to appease even the most skeptical. It was certainly a pleasure to have Dr. Brown take part of my Complementary Medicine Curriculum of 2002.

Sincerely,

Tanya Edwards, MD

Tanya Edwards, MD
Assistant Professor, Department of Family Medicine
Coordinator, Complementary and Alternative Medical Education
Case Western Reserve University School of Medicine
University Hospitals of Cleveland

Department of Family Medicine
School of Medicine

MAILING ADDRESS
Case Western Reserve University
10900 Euclid Avenue
Cleveland, Ohio 44106-4950

Phone 216-844-3791
Fax 216-844-3799

THE FOUNDATION FOR HOLISTIC HEALTH THERAPY

PRESENTS
SEMINARS OF LYMPHATIC MASSAGE

__RAMACHI__ - This is a unique combination of TaiChi and Lymphatic Massage which creates a dynamic self help technique. Includes video tape. 1 day - 4 hours

$99.00

__HEAD AND NECK COURSE__ - Instruction in head and neck technique of Lymphatic Massage. This technique, while confined to the head and neck, affects the entire lymphatic system. Includes video tape. 1 day - 8 hours

$250.00

The following seminars will encompass procedures of both the French and German techniques of Lymphatic Massage. Each 3 day seminar is a total of 25 hours. Completion of any of these courses will be recognized by the Associated Bodywork & Massage Professionals (ABMP) towards eligibility for membership in their national association.

__BASIC COURSE__ - Instruction in the techniques of grounding, centering, and basic techniques of lymphatic drainage. These are combined for a whole body approach to Lymphatic Massage and also include the energetic aspects of the lymphatic arts. Includes student textbook, charts and video tape of the technique.

Dr. William N. Brown is approved by the National Certification Board for Therapeutic Massage and Bodywork (NCBTMB) as a continuing education Approved Provider.

$750.00

__INTERMEDIATE COURSE__ - Perfection of basic techniques and the energies of Lymphatic Massage, also extensive review. Includes instruction on RamaChi, a self help method of Lymphatic Massage. Excellent preparation for the advanced course.

$600.00

__ADVANCED COURSE I__ - Instruction includes techniques for more specific problems including, but not limited to, sinuses, dental afflictions, etc. Includes student textbook.

$500.00

__ADVANCED LYMPHATIC PROTOCOLS– 2 DAYS/12 HRS.__ Whatever style of Lymph Therapy you may have learned, this will make your lymph drainage better! (Pre-approval required)

$295.00

LEARN ADVANCED LYMPHATIC A.L.P.

Discover a dynamic new approach to lymph immune system, health and stress reduction. A.L.P. (Advanced Lymphatic Protocols) created by Dr. William N. Brown, is quick and easy to learn and easy to apply for the betterment of all who may be touched by you.

What are Advanced Lymphatic Protocols?

THEY ARE A METHOD OF CIRCULATORY NUTRITION AND WASTE ELIMINATION THAT WILL BE A PROFOUND BENEFIT FOR THOSE WHO TOUCH WITH SKILL AND COMPASSION AND FOR ALL THOSE WHO ARE TOUCHED AND IN NEED OF HEALTH AND BALANCE

GERIATRIC BENEFIT THRU LUBRICATION OF THE SYNOVIAL JOINTS. A.L.P. HELPS WITH JOINT PROBLEMS AND ARTHRITIS

PROVIDES A PROFOUND STATE OF RELAXATION AND HELPS ELIMINATE STRESS

INCREASES NUTRITION TO SKIN, BALANCES HORMONES, BALANCES NEUROTRANSMITTERS IN BRAIN (INCREASE IN THE UPTAKE OF SEROTONIN) THEREBY HELPING WITH DEPRESSION AND FATIGUE

HELPS MAINTAIN OCULAR PRESSURE IN THE EYE

GENERAL DETOX OF THE BODY AND HELPS ELIMINATE PAIN

How do Advanced Lymphatic Protocols work?

IN A.L.P. YOU WILL LEARN TO OPEN THE LYMPH GATES IN PROPER SEQUENCE ENHANCING AND ACCELERATING THE FLOW OF THE LYMPHATIC SYSTEM AS WELL AS A UNIQUE HEAD AND NECK LYMPHATIC PROCEDURE THAT WILL INCREASE THE FLOW OF THE LYMPH FOR YOUR PATIENT OR LOVED ONE. OPENING THESE GATES ALONG WITH THE PROPER LYMPHATIC PUMPING TO DETOXIFY THRU THE KIDNEYS FACILITATES AND INCREASES THE FLOW OF THE LYMPH STREAM AND SUPPORTS A GENTLE YET THROUGH DETOXIFICATION. WITHOUT THE PROPER SEQUENTIAL OPENING OF THE LYMPH GATES COMBINED WITH THE DETOX PUMP EVEN THOUGH THE LYMPH SYSTEM MAY BE STIMULATED, THE FLOW OF THE LYMPH STREAM WILL NOT BE INCREASED BEYOND AEROBIC ACTIVITY AT 15-20 LITERS OF LYMPH IN ONE HOUR. HOWEVER, WITH THE ADVANCED LYMPHATIC PROTOCOLS THE RATE OF THE FLOW OF THE LYMPH MAY BE INCREASED TO 40 TO 50 LITERS OF LYMPH IN ONE HOUR WITH NO SIGNS OF TOXIC LETHARGY

Why would you want to include A.L.P. in your caregiving program?

1. IT IS QUICK AND EASY
2. EFFECTIVE
3. PAINLESS
4. FACILIATES THE EFFECTIVENESS OF OTHER MODALITIES
5. PATIENTS HEAL FASTER AND QUICKER
6. STRENGTHENS THE IMMUNE SYSTEM WITH ALL THE ATTEND BENEFITS OF STRONGER IMMUNE SYTEM I.E.: FASTER RECOVERY TIMES, LESS SEVERITY OF ILLNESS, LESS ILLNESS

Who can learn A.L.P.?

ANYBODY, EVERYBODY, ITS QUICK, ITS EASY, ITS FUN

MOST FUN IS SEEING THE PROFOUND RESULTS

PATIENTS REMAIN CLOTHED, CAN BE DONE EITHER SEATED OR LYING DOWN

PERFECT FOR ALL CAREGIVERS – THERAPISTS, NURSES, CNA's, HOSPICE PROVIDERS, FAMILY MEMBERS

LEARN IN ONLY TWO DAYS, GO HOME WITH A SKILL

You make a difference, now make it better.

THE FOUNDATION FOR HOLISTIC HEALTH THERAPY

PRESENTS SEMINARS

INTERNATIONALLY/WORLDWIDE

Instructor: Dr. William N. Brown, Ph.D., N.D., L.M.T.

STUDY THE SPIRITUAL, ENERGETIC AND IMMUNE STRENGTHENING SYSTEM OF

LYMPHATIC MASSAGE

-a white light technique-

SEMINARS ON LYMPHATIC MASSAGE

• BASIC COURSE • INTERMEDIATE COURSE • ADVANCED COURSE
• RAMACHI • CELLULITE • LYMPHEDEMA

Instructions on the principals of body mechanics and movement are incorporated into the course taught in the classroom, contained in the text and on video.

*Dr. Brown teaches seminars internationally/worldwide and is available for seminars in your area. Cost of a 3 day BASIC seminar is $750.00 per student ; video tapes, charts and student textbook are available for purchase. (There is no prerequisite for the basic course).

Dr. William N. Brown is approved by the National Certification Board for Therapeutic Massage and Bodywork (NCBTMB) as a continuing education Approved Provider.

* The DVD includes detailed teaching instructions for the precise execution of each movement of the Full Body Technique of Lymphatic Massage. It contains teacher demonstration of the lymphatic technique.

* The charts are a dynamic, efficient schematic of the vortexian induced vector flow in the lymphatic system.

* The student textbook contains information about the lymphatic system and its importance, nutrition and the immune system, life stream acceleration theory and practice, and clinical research.

LYMPHATIC MASSAGE COURSE
****

White Light Body Work For The New Age

****

INSTRUCTOR – DR. WILLIAM N. BROWN

THIS METHOD
-STRENGTHENS THE IMMUNE SYSTEM –
-CLEANSES THE BODY INTERNALLY-
-PROMOTES PROFOUND STATES OF RELAXATION-

LYMPHATIC MASSAGE IS COMPATIBLE WITH ALL OTHER MYOFASCIAL RELEASE TECHNIQUES. THE RESULTS GAINED WITH THIS TECHNIQUE CANNOT BE REPLICATED!

REGISTRATION FORM

Course: Please check appropriate box:

- ☐ **BASIC COURSE**   **$750.00**
- ☐ **INTERMEDIATE COURSE**   **$600.00**
- ☐ **ADVANCED COURSE**   **$500.00**
- ☐ **A.L.P. COURSE**   **$295.00**
- ☐ **RAMA CHI**   **$ 99 .00**

Course Date: _____

Course Location: _____

Name**:** _____

☐ M.D., ☐ P.T., ☐ M.T., ☐ R.N., ☐ Lay Person
(No previous training required for Basic Course)

ADDRESS: _____

CITY: _____   STATE _____

ZIP: _____   HOME PHONE: _____

WORK PHONE: _____   E-MAIL _____

FOR FURTHER INFORMATION, PLEASE CALL
928-282-5517

BOOK, VIDEO TAPES & CHARTS ON LYMPHATIC MASSAGE

1. THE TOUCH THAT HEALS, THE ART OF LYMPHATIC MASSAGE, THE SECRET KEY TO STRENGTHENING THE IMMUNE SYSTEM - A definitive book on the history, technique and practice of lymphatic massage. The book includes the protocols, application and complete instruction with photos on the lymphatic massage technique, including new and incisive theories on AID's causes and prevention, also nutritional lymphatic cleansing recipes, herbs and foods and a newly updated extensive reference on lymphatic massage therapy along with the introduction of ALP (Advanced Lymphatic Protocols).

$49.95

2. RAMACHI - SELF HELP LYMPHATIC MASSAGE -

A video demonstration and instruction of the technique and its relationship to TaiChi by Dr. Brown and Rama Jon.

$29.95

3. INTERVIEWS WITH DR. BROWN - Dr. Brown lectures, interviews, and demonstrations on this entertaining and informative video.

$34.95

4. LECTURE - THE INTERRELATIONSHIP OF NUTRITION AND LYMPHATIC MASSAGE - This DVD includes Dr. Brown's full lecture on the interrelationship of nutrition and Lymphatic Massage and questions from the participants with Dr. Brown's answers.

$34.95

5. HEAD AND NECK TECHNIQUE - SEMINAR - This DVD includes detailed teaching instructions for the precise execution of each movement of the Head and Neck Technique of the Lymphatic Massage. It includes teacher demonstrations of the lymphatic technique. It also includes two interviews with Dr. Brown, his lecture on lymphatic dynamics and questions from the students and participants with Dr. Brown's answers.

$44.95

6. CHARTS - A dynamic, efficient schematic of the vortexian induced vector flow in the lymphatic system. Set of 2 charts.

$25.00

ORDER FORM

ITEM	UNIT PRICE	#ORDERED	TOTAL
Book The Touch that Heals	$49.95	_____	_____
DVD's			
1. RamaChi - Self Help Lymphatic Massage	$29.95	_____	_____
2. Interviews w/Dr. Brown	$34.95	_____	_____
3. Lecture - The Interrelation-ship of Nutrition and Lymphatic Massage	$34.95	_____	_____
4. Head and Neck Technique Seminar	$44.95	_____	_____
Charts			
Set of 2	$25.00	_____	_____

Total Items Ordered: _____ *Shipping & Handling: _____

TOTAL ENCLOSED: $ _____

Name _____

Address _____

City _____ State _____

Zip Code _____ Telephone # _____

*Please include $10.00 per item for shipping & handling. Send cash, money order or personal check only, to: **Dr. William N. Brown, Ph.D., 60 Buena Vista Lane, Sedona, AZ 86336**

THE AMERICAN ASSOCIATION OF LYMPHATIC PRACTITIONERS

Dear Practitioner:

This letter is you invitation to experience membership in a new association. The American Association of Lymphatic Practitioners (AALP). The AALP is a holistic organization dedicated to creating opportunity for its members by providing a supportive environment for the advancement of the practice of lymphatics. This support will be primarily through advertising, networking, referrals, teaching seminars, workshops, research, case histories and field studies.

By becoming a member of the AALP, you will help to ensure the successful mainstream integration of lymphatic modalities throughout the United States. Lymphatic Practitioners include, but are not limited to, anyone who practices manual lymph drainage, lymphatic massage, lymphatic massage, lymphatic energy workers, TaiChi and Ch'ikung. Membership would also be open to doctors, chiropractors, acupuncturists, physical therapists, massage therapists and other health and wellness specialists who have specialized training in the field of lymphatics.

You will be registered as a Lymphatic Practitioner and may use the initials R. L.P. after our name. You will receive a handsome certificate indicating your professional commitment to this specialized field.

You will heighten your therapeutic skills by receiving the **Lymphatic Quarterly**, which will constantly update you on new practices and theories in the national lymphatic community. You will be offered discounts on advertising, educational opportunities and seminars, nationwide.

You can make a difference. Be a part of an organization of competent caring individuals, who are working in the forefront of manual medicine with the most important system in the human physiology, the immune system.

Fill out the application form and send $25.00 (this represents a 50% discount for the first year) for a one year membership to: The Foundation for Holistic Health Therapy, 60 Buena Vista Lane, Sedona, AZ 86336, USA. Attention: AALP. Upon acceptance you will be eligible to networking and referrals.

Yours in health and love,

William N. Brown, Ph.D., N.D., L.M.T.
President/Executive Director
E-mail: drbrown@thetouchthatheals.com
Website: www.thetouchthatheals.com

THE AMERICAN ASSOCIATION OF LYMPHATIC PRACTITIONERS

MEMBERSHIP APPLICATION

NAME _____

ADDRESS _____

CITY _____ STATE _____ ZIP _____

PHONE (H) _____ (W) _____ SS# _____

BIRTHDATE _____ SEX _____

YEARS IN PRACTICE _____

Please attach detailed educational background and training. Include any specialized training in <u>lymphatic modalities.</u>

Send completed application and $25.00 for a one year membership along with a check payable to Dr. William N. Brown to:

> THE FOUNDATION FOR HOLISTIC HEALTH THERAPY
> 60 BUENA VISTA LANE
> SEDONA, AZ 86336
>
> Attention: AALP

PLEASE NOTE: **The Lymphatic Quarterly** is free with an AALP membership. If you would like to subscribe without membership, please send $40.00 for a one year subscription, along with your name and address to the above address.

For information regarding advertising rates, please call (928)-282-5517

INDEX OF CHARTS AND FIGURES

APPENDIX

1. Vodder, Dr. Emil, <u>Manuel Lymph Drainage</u>

2. "Lymph Drainage as Auxiliary Therapy", Lecture read by Dr. G. Gutman, M.D. at the First Congress of International Federation of Manual Medicine, London, September, 1965.

3. Dr. Lieberman, Ph.D., et al., "Mood, Carbohydrates, and Obesity", <u>American Journal of Clinical Nutrition</u>, 1986 p. 46.

4. Dr. Horwitt, <u>American Journal of Clinical Nutrition</u>, 1986.

5. Dr. Simopolus, <u>American Journal of Clinical Nutrition</u>, 1987.

6. <u>Science News</u>, Vol. 125, p. 362.

7. West, Dr. C. Samuel, <u>The Golden Seven Plus One</u>

8. <u>Introduction to Dr. Vodder's Manual Lymph Drainage</u>, Vol. 1, Basic Course, H. & G. Wittlinger.

9. "Lymphatic Manipulation", Lecture from Dr. Annie Childs, Santa Monica, CA, 1982.

10. <u>Healing Aids Naturally</u>

11. Adaptation from the Monfort Report by Dr. Monfort

12. Samyosa Institute, J.F. Garino, "Dr. Vodder's Lymph Drainage".

13. Alexandersson, Olof <u>Living Water</u>

14. Foster, <u>What Really Causes AIDS</u>

15. Kroger, Hanna, <u>God Helps Those Who Help Themselves</u>

16. Horowitz, Leonard G., <u>AIDS, Ebola and Emerging Viruses</u>

17. Horowitz, Leonard G., <u>Death in the Air: Globalism, Terrorism & Toxic Warfare</u>

18. Argüelles, José and Miriam, <u>Mandala</u>

19. Hall, Manley P., <u>The Secret Teachings of All Ages</u>

20. Stone, Randolph, <u>Polarity</u>

21. <u>Physiology and Anatomy Coloring Book</u>

THE FOUNDATION FOR HOLISTIC HEALTH THERAPY, LLC.

SCHOOL OF LYMPHATIC MASSAGE

SEDONA, ARIZONA

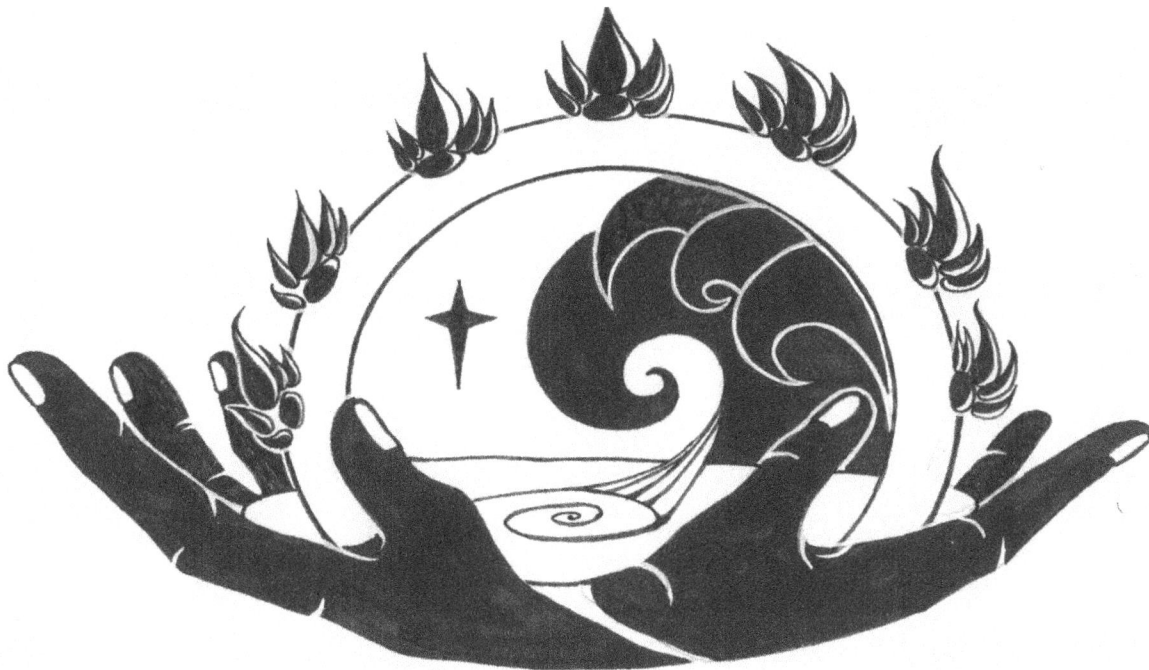

DR. WILLIAM N. BROWN, Ph.D., N.D., D.Sc., L.M.T.

Principal Instructor
in
The Art of Lymphatic Massage

www.ingramcontent.com/pod-product-compliance
Lightning Source LLC
Chambersburg PA
CBHW080241270326

41926CB00020B/4325